PROMETHEUS
AND THE LIVER
THROUGH ART AND MEDICINE

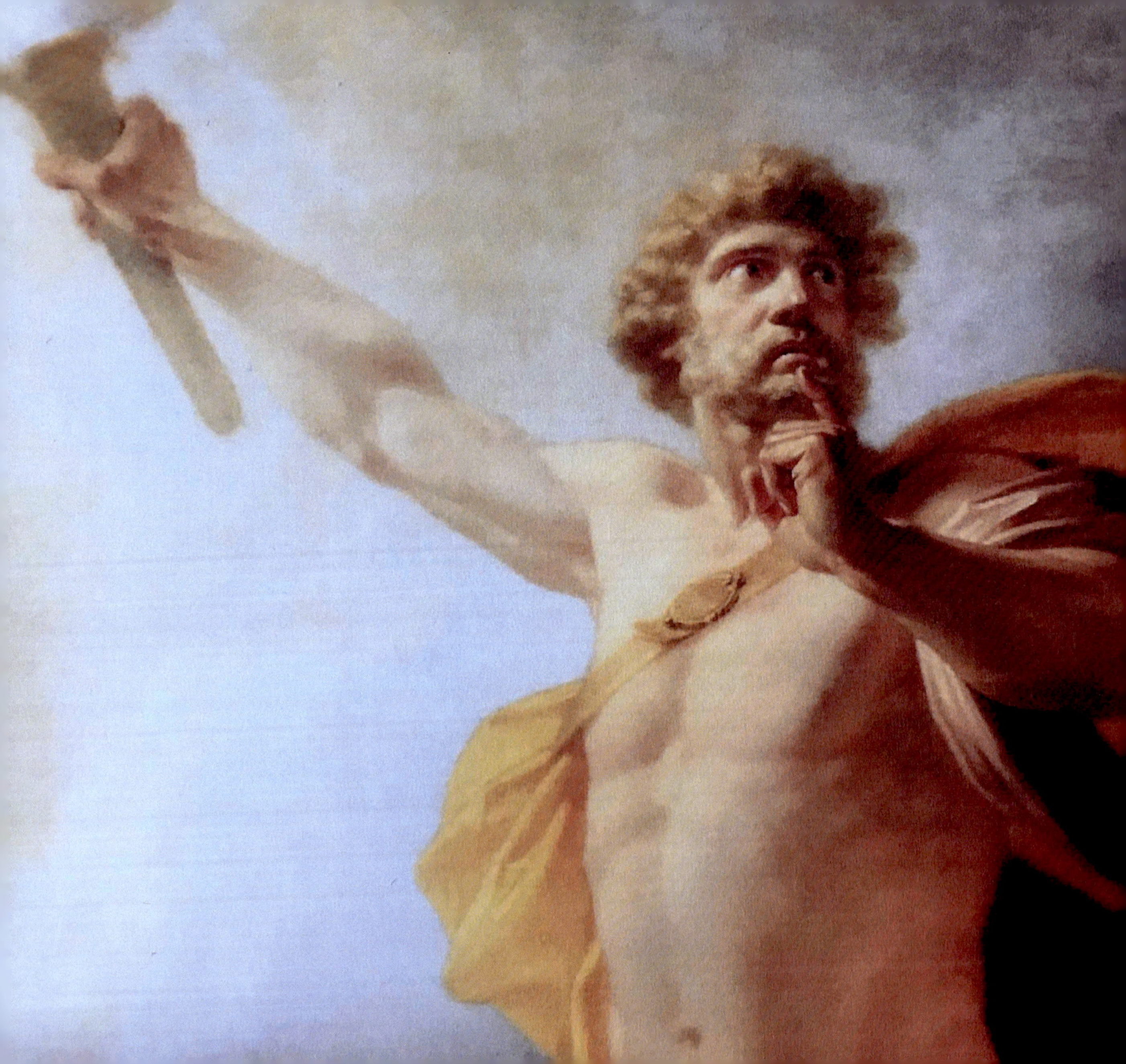

PROMETHEUS AND THE LIVER
THROUGH ART AND MEDICINE

JULIA VAN ROSMALEN, MEREL VAN GULIK,
BELLE VAN ROSMALEN AND THOMAS VAN GULIK

Routledge
Taylor & Francis Group
LONDON AND NEW YORK

CONTENTS

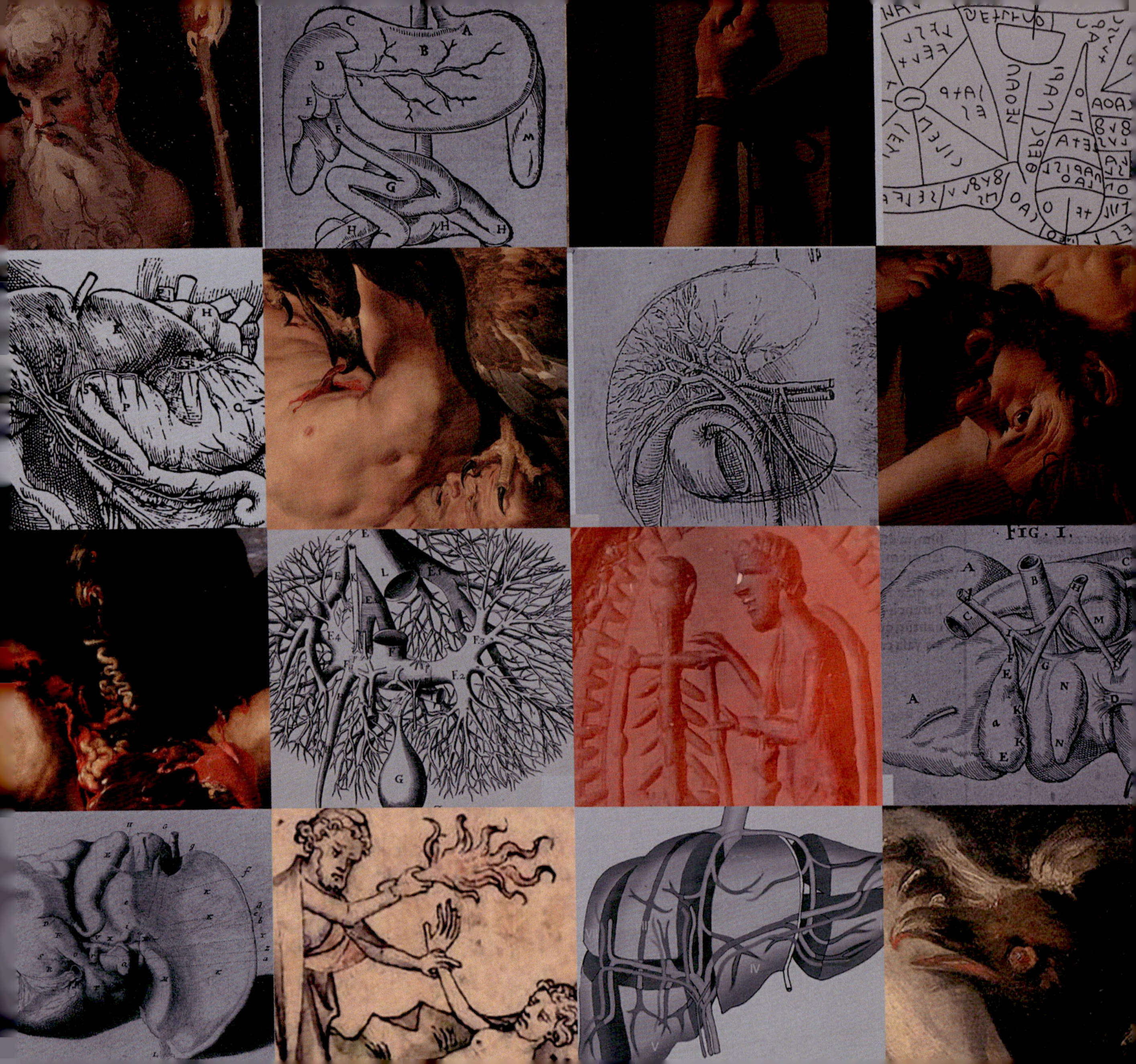
FIG. I.

INTRODUCTION

Prometheus is a figure that has acquired the status of 'martyr' for the human intellect and development. His suffering has been the subject of a large variety of artworks through the ages remaining present in artistic conventions on martyrdom and mythology. Chained to the scraggy precipice of the Caucasus Mountains, Prometheus is visited daily by an eagle that tears out parts of his liver, a practice and punishment that continues into eternity. This endlessness is not solely the result of Prometheus' immortality; the suffering continues because the Titan's liver grows back each night. What crime warrants such a grave punishment for the Titan?

The Greek myth tells us that, during the life of Prometheus, mankind was new--not fully developed nor evolved for life on Earth. These humans had no technical skills, and vitally, no knowledge of fire and its elemental power to sustain life. This ignorance as status quo was pleasing to Zeus, the leader of the gods, whose dominion over humanity hinged on an essential power over the elements. Prometheus, however, was a Titan, a preceding race of powerful beings often at war with the Olympian gods, and thus not fully on the same team as them. He was, essentially, a benefactor to mankind and, in some textual variants of the myth, even their creator. Going behind Zeus' back, the Titan stole the fire of the gods and gave it, hidden in a fennel stalk, to humanity. But where a fire starts to burn, it also starts to spread; before long Zeus discovered the Titan's betrayal. The leader of the Olympians was irate about what Prometheus had done, as the gift of fire would not just bring warmth to humanity, but bring them crafts and development as well. Ingenuity was literally ignited and the process of civilization begins. Passion, ambition and drive, all needed for scientific progress are sometimes called 'fire' after all. And so, Zeus chained Prometheus to the rock and sent his eagle upon him.

Nowadays, we might say that the fire of Prometheus burns on in all of us as it continues to spread. It is, perhaps, thanks to Prometheus that humans have continued to expand their scientific and artistic achievements.

Prometheus and his cruel fate inspired countless artists producing many different types of works – statues, drawings, paintings – and across many art historical periods – antiquity, the middle ages, the renaissance, the baroque, modernity and contemporary art. Galleries and museums around the world hold in their collections images that demonstrate how different eras tackled the myth in myriad ways, emphasizing distinct parts of this story.

In antiquity we see the Prometheus myth reinvented in new editions of the text, which prompts variation in visual interpretations of the Titan's story. In the Middle Ages, the myth had to find its position and be embedded in a Christianised worldview in a way that it didn't conflict with the new faith. Here, we often see Prometheus as the creator of mankind, as a parallel to the Christian God. In the Renaissance, we can observe a newfound appreciation for the ancient texts while discovering the Prometheus myth referenced in works by humanist scholars, who included the Titan's story in their complex allegories to showcase their learning and development. In the Baroque, a twofold fascination for dramatic pathos on one side and scientific interest in anatomy on the other, made suffering bodies a favoured subject in art. It comes as no surprise that in this era we find the famous monumental paintings that put the punishment of Prometheus front and centre in compositions that demonstrate both a sublime suffering and a medicalization of death; the eagle acts as a surgeon, seemingly giving the beholder an anatomy lesson as it tears out the Titan's liver. With the advent of modernity, there is an increased literary fascination in Prometheus and his story. The myth inspired famous poets like Johann Wolfgang von Goethe and Percy Byshe Shelley, for whom the Titan became an embodiment of the Romantic ideal. Mary Shelley, the latter poet's wife, gives an original and subversive spin on the Prometheus myth in her novel *Frankenstein: the Modern Prometheus*. Across all media, Prometheus serves as an inspiration for artists, authors, and composers—such as Beethoven and Schubert—alike. The focus drifts away from an 'accurate' or strictly textual representation of the myth towards a more personal connection between artist and the Titan and what his suffering represents. This shift intensifies in the twentieth century, where art movements followed each other in swift succession and a large variety of artists used Prometheus as a symbol, now almost completely isolated from its myth, in order to communicate their vastly different and sometimes directly contrasting ideologies. The changing approaches to the depiction of the myth through the ages mirrors the zeitgeists that influenced developments in medical practice, with the organ of the liver being the point of connection between the two.

In Greek mythology, the liver was seen as the seat of life, the central organ in both gods and men, to which religious and mystical properties were attributed. It was also the organ used by soothsayers too predict the future, which they could 'read' in the protuberances in a sheep's liver. Today, we understand the liver to be a complex organ with several essential functions for the biological processes of metabolism and digestion. Liver failure is not compatible with life and we cannot – despite all our modern medical and technical advancements – replicate its functions artificially. So, did the ancient Greeks also imagine life, even the life of an immortal one, to be impossible without a liver? If this were so, Prometheus would not survive his punishment. But, the Titan's curse is, essentially, that his liver regenerates overnight, ready to be destroyed again at the eagle's daily visit. This could be due to Prometheus immortal nature, causing lost parts of the body to regenerate, a property found more often in Greek myth. In a similar vein as the Hydra of

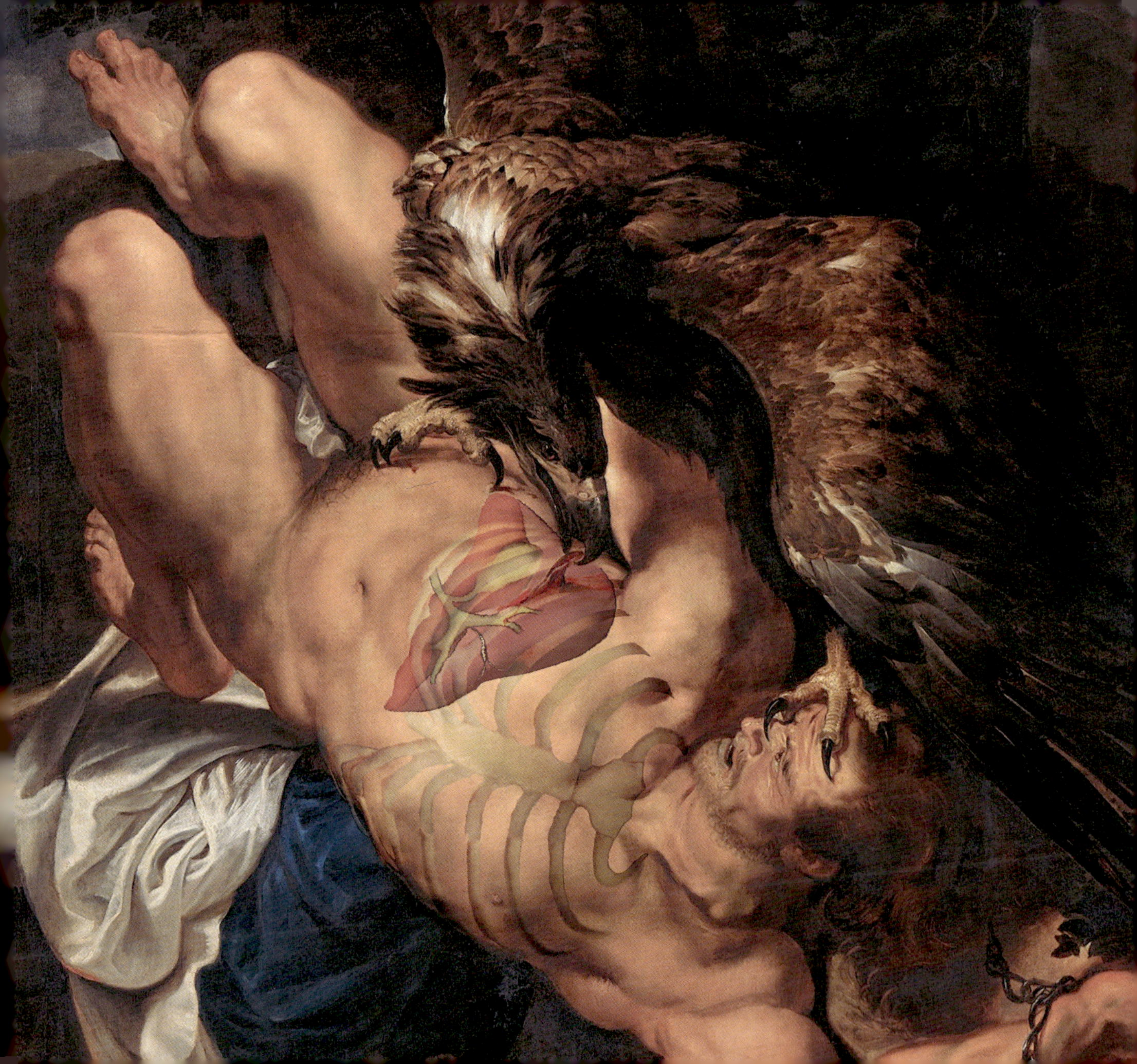

Lerna, a nine-headed serpentine monster where the cutting off of one head prompted the regeneration of not one, but even two heads.

It has only been in the last few decades that scientists have documented the fact that the liver does have actual regenerative properties. This process can be observed after the loss of part of the liver, which is then compensated for by the organ, which slowly regrows that lost part. This is a property that is largely relied upon by surgeons nowadays when surgery calls for the removal of part of the liver. Not the eagle, but the scalpel removes the liver, and the organ faithfully regenerates. To many surgeons and doctors, this property has made Prometheus the symbol, or patron, of liver surgery.

In the development of the field of medicine, each era possesses its own view on the liver and the role the organ fulfils within the human body, in accordance to current medical knowledge and social practices. This book gives an overview of these developments, looking at the long history of the liver and its known properties, while simultaneously tracing depictions of Prometheus through art history. What did artists, audiences and patrons learn about the appearance and functions of this organ when they saw it being devoured by the eagle in artworks, and what significance did the liver have for them?

The liver is of crucial importance for health and wellbeing. Because of this, scientific research in the last few decades has produced significant successes in the treatment of afflictions of the liver. Prometheus' Olympic fire, that he brought to mankind, was one of the advent of knowledge, and thus of progress. It is also in this sense that Prometheus is a symbol for the ambition of medical professionals working in research when they strive to improve the treatment of liver related illnesses. Like Prometheus they aim to look ahead and explore the new frontiers of treatment.

In *Prometheus and the liver through art and medicine*, the figure of Prometheus is investigated in a threefold approach. First, the Titan's role in Greek mythology is expanded upon: we feature a brief retelling of his story of how Prometheus stole the fire and brought it to mankind and how Zeus subsequently punished him for this act. Secondly, he is viewed through the lens of the visual arts. We give an overview of the most prominent works of art that illustrate the myth of Prometheus and especially, his punishment. Lastly, we trace the development of medical knowledge on the liver, and place these advancements within art historical timelines. Here, pioneers in medicine and scientists will be featured who, in a manner akin to Prometheus, sought to transgress the boundaries of knowledge. Their gift to humanity was medical advancement, in order to better understand the organ and its function. The phenomenon of regeneration is one of the most fascinating properties of the liver. And it is the study of this property that motivated technical advancements in the field of liver surgery from the twentieth century onward. Groundbreaking surgeries such as resection of part of the liver, or the removal of the entire liver which was then replaced by a donor organ, were conceptualised and put into practice. Prometheus and his tortured liver were well avenged by these procedures that followed from his gift of fire, which becomes a gift of knowledge.

Fig. 0.1 Prometheus Bound, Reception piece for the French Royal Academy, 1762, Marble statue, 114 cm x 82 cm x 48 cm, Musée du Louvre, Paris

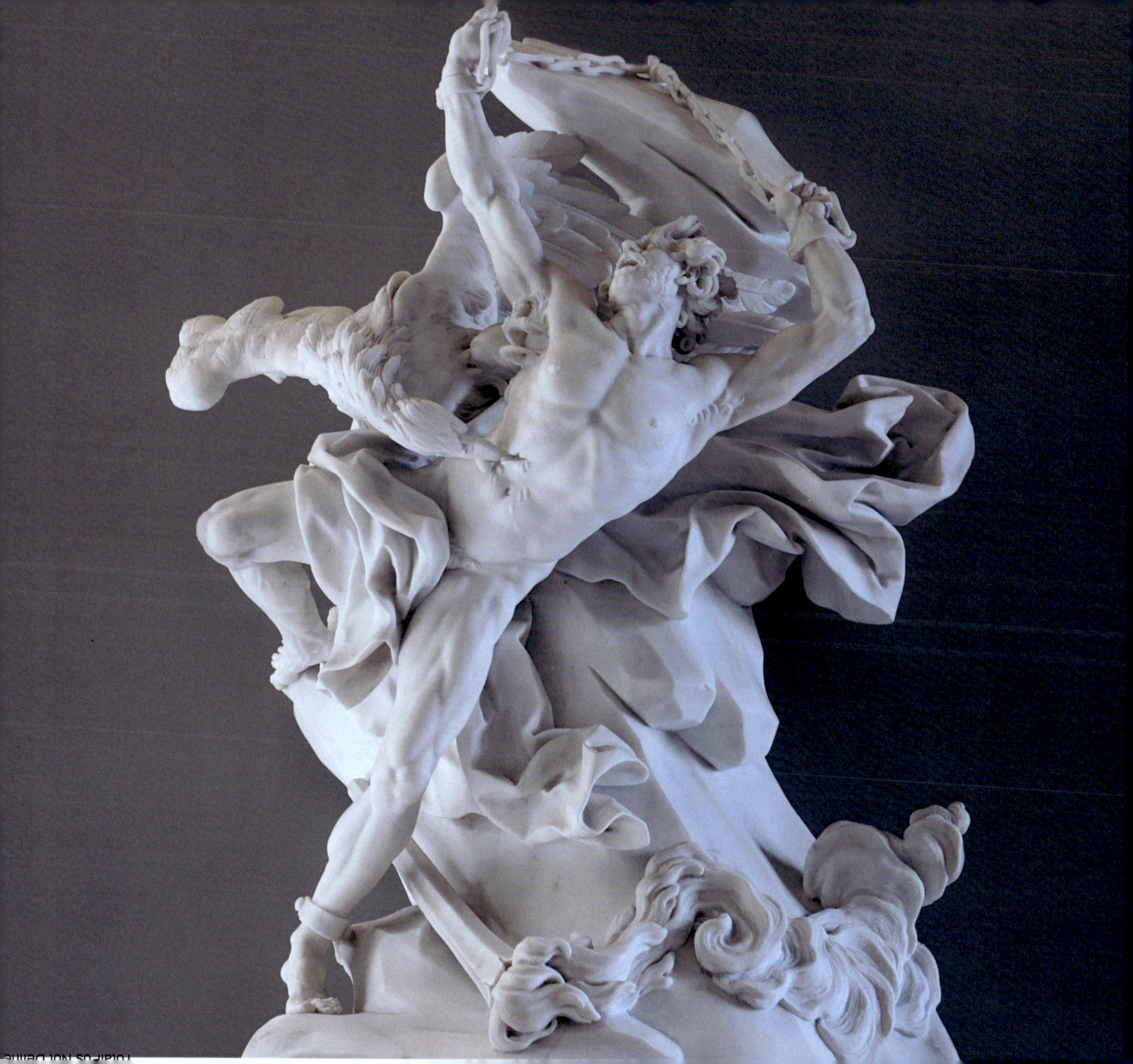

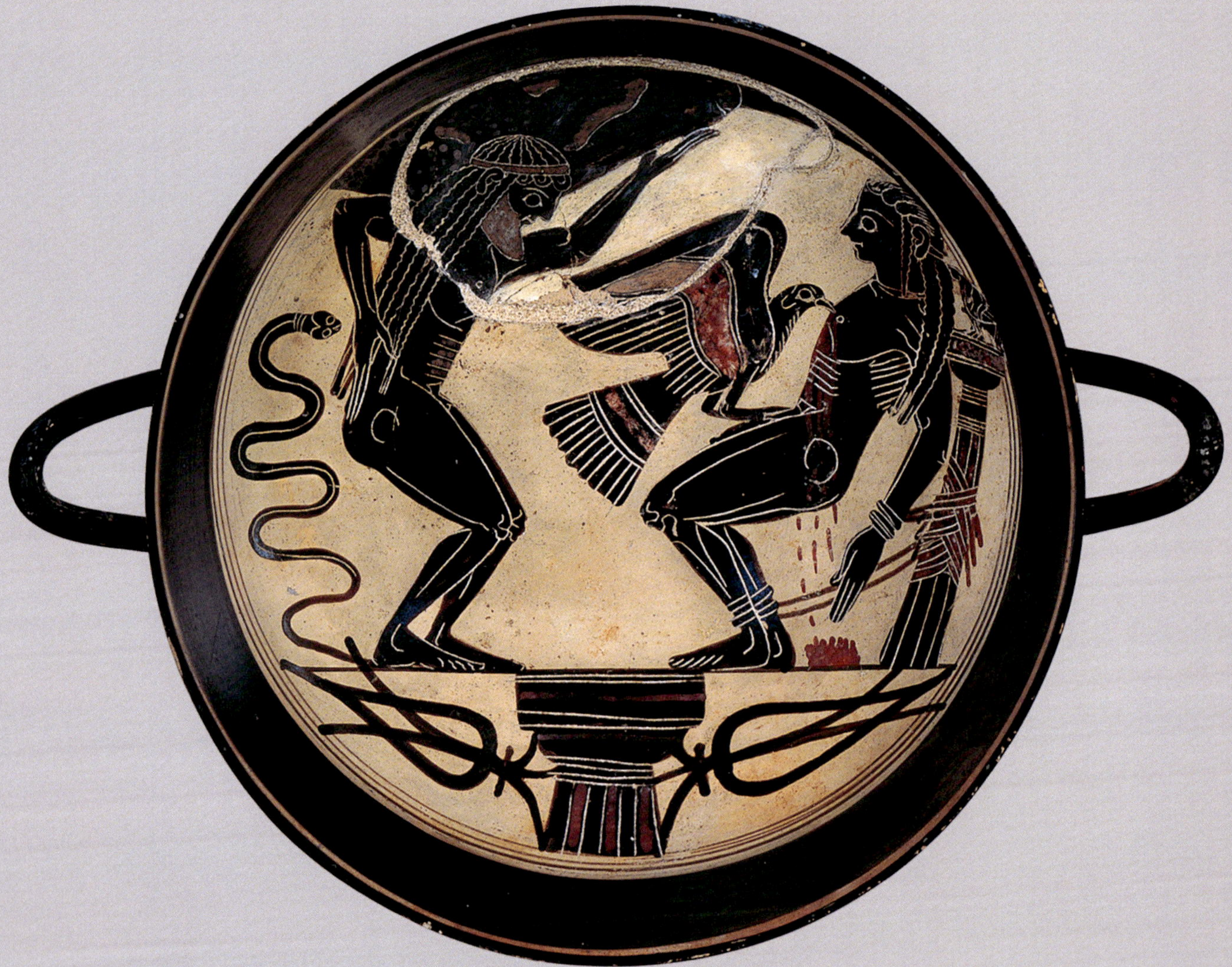

1
THE PROMETHEUS MYTH

PROMETHEUS AND EPIMETHEUS

Prometheus wasn't human. Yet his story is as benefactor to mankind. The hero was a Titan – one of the twelve pre-Olympic gods that were the direct offspring of the primordial deities Gaia, mother earth, and Uranus, god of the sky. When the Olympic gods decided to create mankind, they asked Prometheus – 'He who looks ahead' (προ / pro – before, μανθάνω / mantháno – thinking, understanding) – and his brother, Epimetheus – 'The thinker of the afterthought' (επι / epi – after) – to provide humans and animals with the correct characteristics. Epimetheus asked if he could divide these properties over

Fig. 1.1 Ancient Greek bowl with depiction of Prometheus, chained to a column, is visited by an eagle who, during the day, tears out a large part of his liver. In the night the liver regrows. Left we see Atlas, the brother of Prometheus, who carries the heavens on his shoulders. The snake behind him is Ladon, a serpentine dragon that guards the golden apples in the garden of the Hesperides. The mountain Atlas and the Caucasus mountains were regarded as the edges of the world by the ancient Greeks. Laconic kylix with Prometheus and Atlas, 560-550 BCE, 20,2 x 14,4 cm, Collection Vatican Museum, Rome

the living creatures and his brother agreed. As Prometheus watched his brother work, he noticed that he had saved humans for last and there were barely any properties left: no claws, no fur, no fangs, and no tools. Panicked by the disadvantage this division would place upon humans, Prometheus decided to give them the fire of the Olympic god Hephaistos and simultaneously, the craftiness of Athena—a trait relayed through the theft.

PROMETHEUS CREATES HUMANS OUT OF CLAY

In a different version of the myth from later antiquity and especially prevalent in Rome, Prometheus was the one to create mankind at Zeus's request. The Titan sculpted figurines in different colours out of clay and Aphrodite joined him to bring them to life with her breath. Prometheus helped the humans – only men so far – and provided for them, all to Zeus' contentment. Yet, Prometheus couldn't shake the feeling that there had to be more to this: the life of the humans was so dull, so monotonous...nothing was happening! Every day was the exact same as the one that came before. The humans weren't aware of any other kind of life and thus had no experience of trouble. Prometheus, on the other hand, knew exactly what was lacking: fire. But he was also aware that Zeus would be absolutely unwilling to share that element with mankind, as it would make them feel so powerful that they would refuse to honour him. Because the Titan understood this condition, he left the humans in their natural, ignorant state for a considerable period.

PROMETHEUS BRINGS HUMANS THE OLYMPIC FIRE

Until one day, Prometheus couldn't stand by idly anymore. Humans needed fire in order to discover new things: to build, to eat... to dare to think, or take risks. To his great shock, Prometheus heard Zeus say that he might destroy the humans on a whim. How could those poor helpless creatures ever defend themselves against such action? If they had the fire, they could at least defend themselves. Prometheus decided to take fate into his own hands and to steal the fire from Hephaistos, the smith of Olympus and his distant cousin. He chose a moment where Zeus would be enjoying an elaborate feast and thus wouldn't notice the theft.

Armed with a fennel stalk, which was known in antiquity for matchstick-like properties, he snuck into Hephaistos' smithy on the mountain precipice at the backside of Olympus. To his shock he found Brontes, one of the Cyclopes employed by Hephaistos, still present in the smithy. Thankfully the being was asleep. Prometheus extended his fennel stalk and held it in the fire, catching the flame and triumphantly returned to the humans on Earth.

Initially the sight of the fire frightened and perplexed the humans. How could they be experiencing light and warmth when the sun had already gone down? It was as if the sun had been brought to earth in the hands of Prometheus. When Prometheus saw them hide in fear, he spoke to them: "Don't be frightened! This will greatly improve your lives." When the humans saw the kind eyes in the face of their benefactor whom they trusted so well, they realised they had to overcome their fear and learn more about this new element. This pleased Prometheus, who felt assured that he had done a good deed. Immediately, he started teaching the humans the basics of keeping a fire: how to keep it burning, how to make sure you don't get burned, how do you roast meat or fish, how to cook the perfect egg...

ZEUS AND THE SACRIFICIAL MEATS, THE TRICK AT MECONE

In his book *Work and days*, the Greek poet Hesiodos included a different reason for Prometheus' theft. The poet narrates that Zeus had decided that the humans should bring sacrifices to the gods, arranging a meeting at Mecone so that the habitants of Mount Olympus could agree on the nature of the gift: what parts of the sacrificial animal would belong to the gods, and what parts to the humans. Prometheus helped the humans prepare two plates: on one, he put all the good meat and organs, but he covered it up with the grotesque stomach of the ox; on the other, he placed all the leftover bones and inedible pieces, but covered it with appealing, appetizing glistening fat. When Zeus was invited to choose which of the plates he would prefer in offering, he was misled, chosing the dish covered in glistening fat. When the god discovered this deception, he was enraged, taking fire away from the humans as punishment. It is clear that in this version of the myth, humans already had and were aware of fire and its properties. Prometheus, in his guilt, steals the fire back from Olympus for mankind, an act that only serves to further engender the wrath of Zeus.

THE REVENGE OF ZEUS

Zeus had barely begun his dessert when he noticed something strange. It was well past sundown, yet there seemed to be light on Earth in the human settlements at the foot of Olympus. When he looked closer, he discovered there wasn't just one fire, but countless small fires and lamps. Standing over the largest flame was Prometheus. The humans were captivated as the Titan told them of the many uses of fire and the endless potential of its application. Zeus immediately understood what had happened; he recalled Prometheus asking him why he didn't want to share the fire with humans. "Because that's the end of everything, Prometheus! The end of my reign," he had answered him. He saw that he hadn't convinced the Titan, but he decided not to argue any further. He knew very well that he would never convince the stubborn Prometheus—the humans were apparently far too dear to him. Zeus regretted that he hadn't been firmer with Prometheus, who seemed to care little about whether or not the supreme god was venerated.

Initially Zeus was furious with Prometheus, but found himself mostly disappointed in his friend. What had started as a fun experiment with clay creatures had turned into a painful disregard of his authority – and for that to come from Prometheus of all people, one of his dear friends. This betrayal was unforgiveable, and an appropriate punishment was in order. Zeus decided that both Prometheus and his beloved humans would have to pay. The humans now enjoyed such an easy life, full of so many benefits and opportunities that it wouldn't be long until they found themselves able to rival the gods, and even try to overthrow them. This was something that needed to be nipped in the bud immediately. Because the humans would, with fire, be able to defend themselves against 'simple' punishments,—and because Prometheus would try to protect them—Zeus would have to match the craftiness of their protector and turn to trickery as well.

Zeus was aware that Prometheus had been disappointed that he had only created men.

So, with that in mind, he asked the Titan to come visit him. Prometheus showed up, tense because he was aware of what he had done, but Zeus completely ignored the entire fire question. Prometheus was surprised but he'd be crazy if he were to bring it up himself! Instead Zeus kept talking about how outstanding his meal had been, especially how surprising the dessert was. "and you know what, Prometheus? I've been thinking lately. I changed my mind; it would be a good idea to introduce women to the humans. However, and I hope you agree with me here, you've already created so much! I think it would be fair if Hephaistos gets to take his turn creating this one."

HEPHAISTOS CREATES THE WOMAN, PANDORA

Prometheus did expect something was up, but he didn't see another choice other than to enthusiastically agree to Zeus' offer. When Hephaistos had finished the figure of the woman, Aphrodite was once again called to breathe life into her, like she had done with the men. Zeus invited the other gods to come visit this woman. One by one, they came to see the newest creation, presenting her with gifts. Athena gave her the aptitude for crafts, the Graces gave her jewellery, Hermes taught her language and the art of lying, and so on. Finally, Zeus named his new creation: Pandora ('all the gifts'). Before she was sent to mankind, he gave her one last gift: a sealed jar. He told her it was a purely decorative object, and that she shouldn't break it nor open it. The god added cunningly, "what does it matter, what's inside it?"

THE MARRIAGE OF EPIMETHEUS AND PANDORA

Prometheus perceived that something bad was about to happen, so he warned his brother Epimetheus to, for the time being, not accept any gifts, "especially if they're coming from Olympus!" Epimetheus nodded in agreement and promised his brother he wouldn't, but Prometheus didn't feel very re-assured, because, let's just say that Epimetheus tended to think *after* he'd already done something.

Barely a day had passed and Hermes appeared on Epimetheus' doorstep, and he wasn't visiting alone: he had brought Pandora with him – a completely bewildering creature for

Epimetheus, who had never seen a woman before. She resembled a goddess, but smaller, and... more lifelike. "Can we come in for a bit Epimetheus? I'd like to introduce you. This is Pandora, your future wife," clever Hermes spoke. Any thoughts about Prometheus' admonition immediately disappeared from Epimetheus' head; he was absolutely enamoured with by Pandora.

They were married and, shortly thereafter, the subject of Pandora's jar was raised. Epimetheus asked his wife about this strange vessel that she always took with her, but never opened. Pandora answered that it was a gift from Zeus, and that the contents didn't matter; but, from that that moment on she couldn't put the thought of the jar out of her head. Why would someone gift her an empty, sealed jar? And if it was empty, why bother sealing it and telling her not to open it? She was determined not to break her promise to Zeus and, in order to banish the thoughts from her head, she decided to bury the jar in the garden.

'HOPE' REMAINS IN PANDORA'S JAR

This brought Pandora some of the reprieve she had hoped for and, for a couple of weeks, she was as happy as a newlywed could possibly be. One night, she had trouble falling asleep. Her thoughts kept wandering to the buried jar. Restlessly, she tossed and turned until she couldn't take it anymore. She got out of bed and walked outside, directly to where she had buried the vessel and dug into the earth with her bare hands. She dug faster and faster, almost taken over by a frenzy, and before she knew it, the jar was open in her hands. She could barely take the time to contemplate what she had done as out of the jar burst a wild storm of creatures. Among the chaos and cacophonous noise, she saw fur, teeth animal wings – bats? – all came flying out of the jar! The stream seemed never ending, only growing in number and size. Epimetheus was startled awake by the noise and, getting out of bed to see what was happening, became paralysed as he stood in the doorway, looking at his wife. Seeing her husband, Pandora snapped out of her trance, trying with all her might to force the jar closed once more. When she finally succeeded, the harm had already been done. The creatures released were all manner of evils: disasters, diseases and worries spread over the earth.

There was only one creature left in the jar: hope. Through the ages, this last part of the story has received different interpretations. A pessimistic interpretation tells us that the inheritance of plagues is the human lot; hope remains trapped in the jar. A slightly more optimistic interpretation is that the Greek word used for 'hope' here (ἐλπίς), should be read as 'expectation' and symbolises 'foresight', especially the ability to foresee disaster. Because ἐλπίς remained in the jar, humans, like Epimetheus before them, will never see disaster coming and always assume the best. A final, and most positive interpretation is that no matter what kinds of disasters befall mankind, we will always have hope.

With these plagues released into the world, a new age dawned, and humans learned to know pain and suffering. Consequently, Zeus decided that this race of men should be exterminated, and sent an all-encompassing flood to destroy Earth. All humans drowned, with exception of the daughter of Pandora and Epimetheus and the son of Prometheus. The two became the ancestors of mankind, of us, and according to this legend, we carry the bloodline of both brothers within ourselves. We possess the naivety and impulsiveness of Epimetheus as well as the foresight of Prometheus.

THE PUNISHMENT OF PROMETHEUS

Zeus witnessed the fruits of his destruction and realised that he shouldn't punish mankind any further. But the god didn't want Prometheus to take away all human hardship for a second time. It was appropriate now that Prometheus receive his punishment. Zeus knew just what to do with the Titan, summoning Prometheus once again, the latter realising that the bell tolled for him. Demurely, he followed Zeus, who brought him to the base of the Caucasus Mountains and ordered him to climb the precipice. When Prometheus had reached the top Zeus spoke to him: "you will be chained here for eternity, with no hope for escape or forgiveness. Every day you shall be visited by an eagle, who will peck out your liver and devour it, and every night it shall regrow (fig. 1.1). You, ironically named 'he who looks ahead', did not see this punishment coming. You don't honour your name!" Prometheus answered with a sad smile: "No, Zeus, I knew this would be my fate, but I carefully deliberated and the future of mankind weighs heavier than my own wellbeing and I made a well-funded decision based on that. I ensured that they will prosper and live on, independent of whichever god." This proclamation only infuriated the leader of the Olympic gods, who pronounced, "you hardly deserve my eagle!"

PROMETHEUS FREED

Years later, Zeus begot a son (with the mortal Alcmene) who he treasured dearly: Herakles. Herakles was punished by Zeus' jealous wife Hera, who resented his birth and ordered her husband's child to complete twelve labours. During one of these tasks, the god's son encountered Prometheus chained to the Caucasus. Moved by his plight, Herakles killed the eagle that tormented the Titan, freeing him from his chains. Zeus didn't intervene; this act of heroic compassion would make his treasured son an even bigger hero when he returned to Earth. And so it happened that after centuries of excruciating punishment, Prometheus was allowed to return to Olympus.

The punishment was, as Prometheus had told Zeus, a form of sacrifice: he put the wellbeing of mankind before his own comfort and safety. It is in this action that we can locate an analogy between the doctors of our day who transgress boundaries to find better treatments for their patients. The connection goes further: without the sacrifice Prometheus made, humans wouldn't have been able to develop to our current levels. We would not be able to discover new things, take risks and deliberate the ends to justify the means, and make personal sacrifices to look ahead. These advances include the doctors that dare to go beyond to find new treatments and inspire their colleagues to follow their example. Prometheus' sacrifice hadn't been in vain: he has been an inspiration and example for scientists and artists, and continues to be so to this day.

Fig. 1.2 Prometheus is freed by Herakles, who is aiming his bow at the eagle. Detail of a fresco from the columbarium of the Villa Doria Pamphili, 30-23 BCE. Museo Nationale Romano, Palazzo Massimo alle Terme, Rome

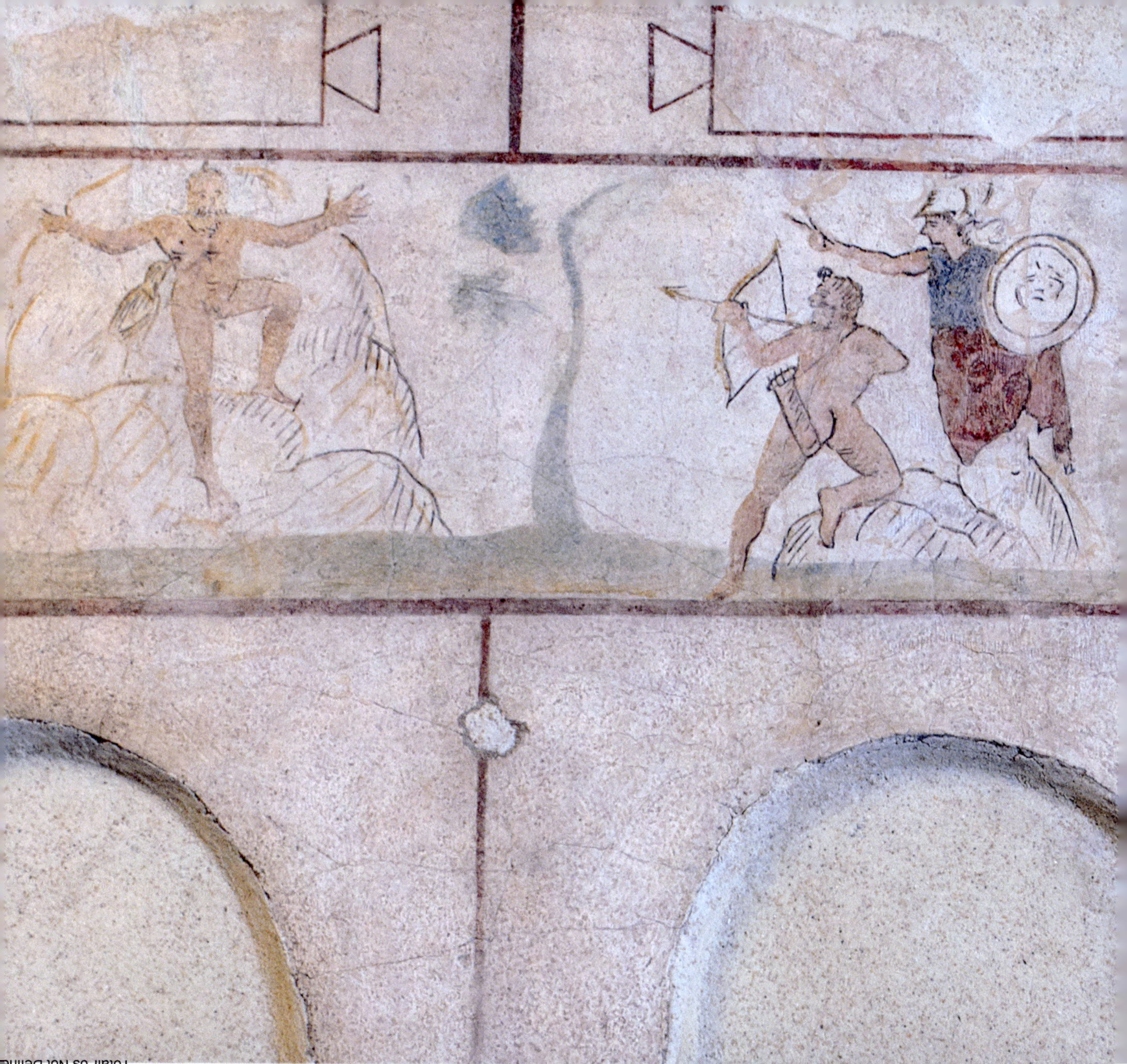

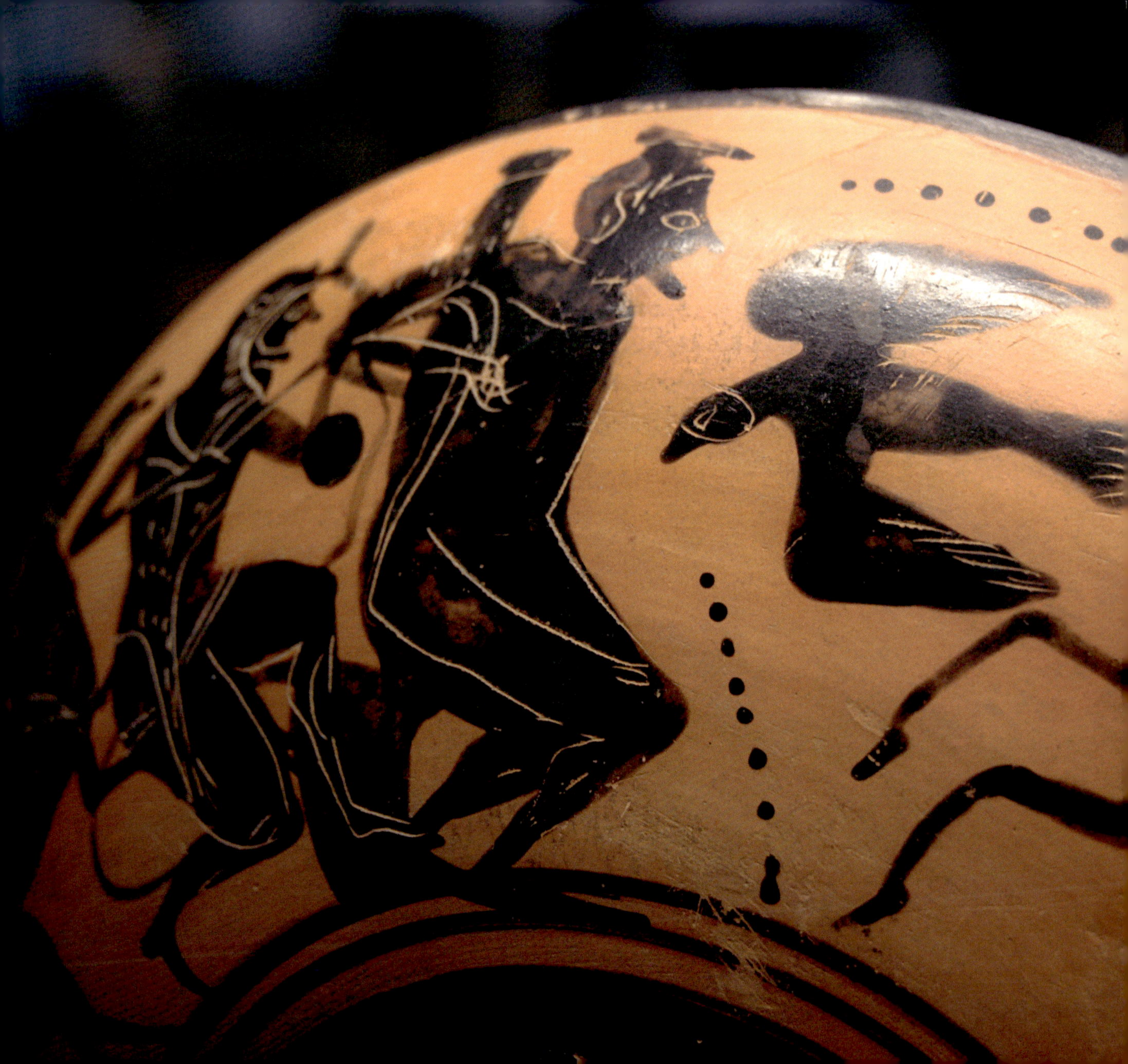

2

THE DEPICTION OF PROMETHEUS IN CLASSICAL ANTIQUITY

The Prometheus myth has been handed down to us through the pens of several different authors. Each of them added to or removed elements of the story, altering the myth and its implications for society. All of these adaptations can be located in the visual arts of classical antiquity. This interplay between text and image is called iconography, and Prometheus' iconographical tradition is rooted in early formal image making and begins at the same time and place as the stories, when the myth was still a 'living' myth. This chapter will examine a selection of the early correspondences between text and artwork.

Afb 2.0 Herakles frees Prometheus, Black figure vase painting on a Beothian cup from Athens, 500 CE, Louvre, Paris

The oldest known written account of the myth is found in the work of Greek poet Hesiodos, who was active between circa 750 to 650 BCE. The myth appears in two of his most important texts: the *Theogony* – which translates to 'origin of the gods' – and *Works and Days*, where the Pandora episode of the myth is told. The *Theogony* relays the Greek Pantheon, the Greek Olympic gods, telling of its origins, and the relations and connections between gods. An important part of this story is the large-scale battle between the Olympian gods and their predecessors, the Titans. Prometheus belonged to the group group of the titans; he functioned as a clever trickster figure that challenged the all-might of Zeus through subterfuge and trickery. In Hesiodos' version of the myth, the function of Prometheus' role is ambiguous: he is a benefactor to the humans, but he is finally bested and condemned by Zeus. The author's own judgment seems to fall in favour of Zeus. As he states that the might of the king of the gods cannot be undermined. Hesiodos relates that the Titan is chained to a pillar when he is visited by the eagle. In a later version by the playwright Aeschylus, he is chained to a rock formation in the Caucasus.

A PREHISTORICAL PROMETHEUS

The earliest known images we have of Prometheus may predate this first record from Hesiodos. This signals a possible, older, oral tradition in which the myth may have been told: a Prometheus story that predates his written history.

One of the earliest known depictions of Prometheus is an ivory plaquette (fig. 2.1) found within the wall of an Archaic temple in Sparta. The plaquette was found amid pottery shards from the geometric period – the oldest period in ancient Greek art defined by geometric patterning on early ceramics. The plaquette shows Prometheus in a contorted kneeling pose, his hands tied to his feet behind his back. He leans backward as the eagle lands on his chest to peck at his

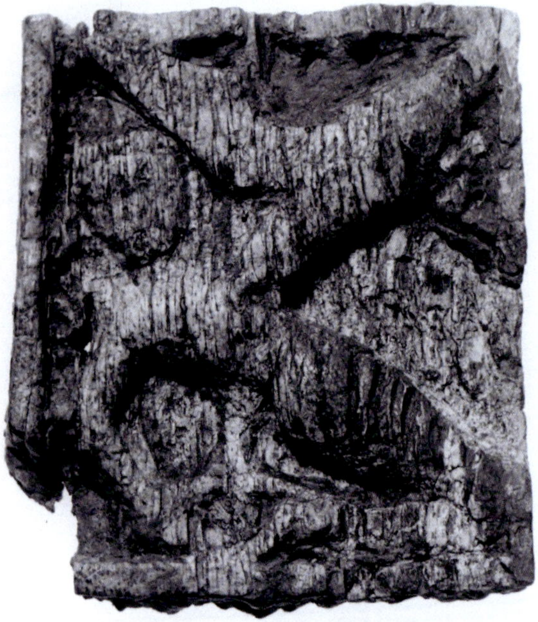

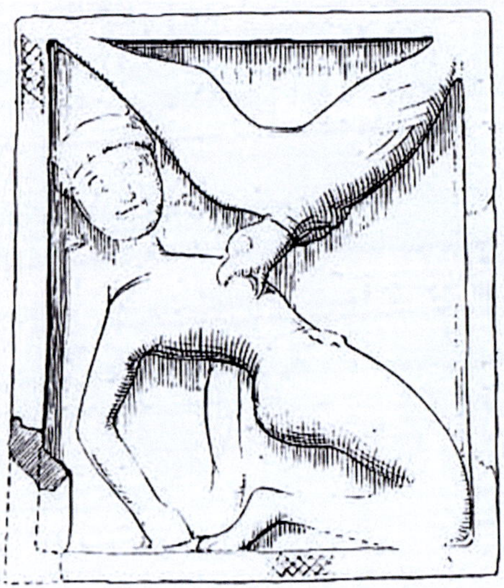

Fig. 2.1 Ivory plaquette where we see Prometheus kneeling down with his hands and feet bound to his back while the eagle tears open his chest. The legs of the eagle have broken off but on his thigh the talons are still visible, digging into his flesh. Late 8th- early 7th century BCE, 7,3 x 6,5 x 1 cm, National Archaeological Museum, Athens.

liver. The legs of the eagle have not survived the passage of time, but traces of the bird's talons are visible on Prometheus' thigh, emphasizing the ruinous nature of the eagle's visits. It is remarkable that this depiction of Prometheus at his punishment possesses neither column nor mountain range on which the Titan is chained; his hands are bound to his feet instead.

A similar scene can be found on a bronze shield ornament from Olympia (Fig 2.2). We find Prometheus with his hands chained behind his back; once again the column or mountain range is absent. In this depiction, the Titan's knees are pulled up in front of him, the eagle flies in from in the upper left corner, approaching menacingly and signalling imminent punishment.

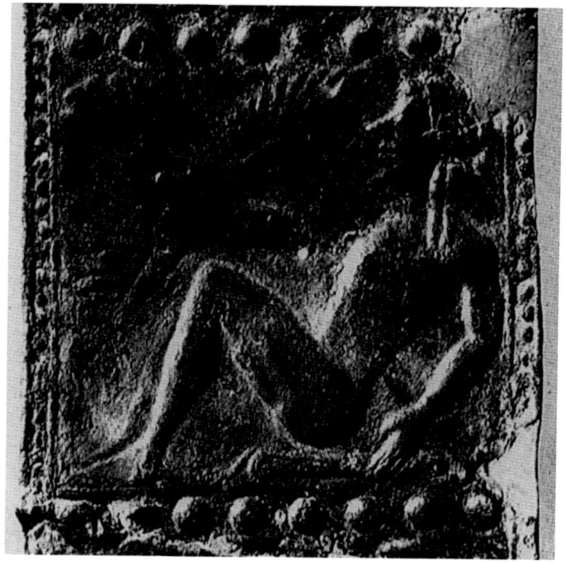

Fig. 2.2 Bronze shield ornament. Prometheus is bound by his hands and feet, with his hands behind his back. The eagle lands on his knees. Archaeological museum of Olympia.

Both of these objects were found on the Peloponnesus and the earliest date proposed for them based on stylistic analysis is the late eight century BCE which means they possibly predate Hesiodos' works. However, both Hesiodos' works and the objects can only receive broad date ranges. Therefore, it can't be said with certainty whether the artists based themselves on the scene as described by Hesiodos or on a preceding story disseminated orally and native to the Peloponnesus. The lack of column and the figure of Herakles – who plays a central role in the myth as told by Hesiodos and figures in later depictions that explicitly reference the poet's adaptation – would grant credibility to the theory that the iconography of these early object comes from an earlier oral tradition. It is also possible that both Hesiodos and these unknown artists drew on the same native oral source.

THE ATTIC PROTOTYPE

The next developments in Promethean iconography can be found in black-figure style vase paintings from Attika. Unlike the earliest objects described above, these depictions

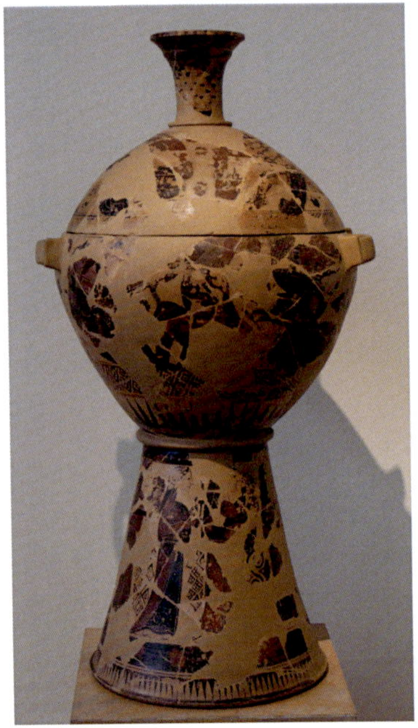

explicitly reference the story as it was described by Hesiodos. One of the first examples of the depiction of Prometheus from this era can be found on a so-called 'skyphos krater', now in the National Archaeological museum in Athens (fig. 2.3). A *skyphos krater* is a type of Greek earthenware vessel with a lid and two handles, elevated on a high foot. This particular *krater* has been reconstructed, —at some point in its history, it shattered into many fragments—but the scenes that once adorned the vase are still recognisable, and indeed, the belly of the vase contained a scene from the Prometheus myth (fig. 2.4). Prometheus is, his hands once again bound behind his back, depicted as the central figure of the setting. In this depiction, he seems to be vertically penetrated by the column. To his left, Herakles kneels, firing his arrows at the eagle approaching from the right side of the composition. Zeus' son's arrows hit their mark and blood is seen flowing from the bird. In addition to the figures, ornamental and highly stylized flowers fill the negative space in the image. This decorative phenomenon is typical for early Greek vase painting and is called 'horror vacui' (dreading the emptiness). The presence of Herakles and the column – which were not found in earlier depictions – illustrate an explicit reference to the Hesiodos text. There are no known contemporaneous examples of this phenomenon elsewhere, so it is likely an Attic invention.

This faithfulness to the text of Hesiodos becomes clear when we compare the Attic *krater* with the bowl in the Vatican Museum featured earlier (fig. 1.1). These two objects illustrate two different artistic readings of the text by Hesiodos. When the poet describes Prometheus' punishment in *Theogony* (lines 520-525), he writes that Zeus chained Pro-

Fig. 2.3 Early black figure, Attic Skyphos krater, discovered in the grave field of Anagyrous (Near Vary, Attica), On the belly of the vase we see Prometheus impaled by a high column, across from him crouches Herakles, ready to shoot the eagle that approaches from Prometheus' other side (see detail in Fig. 2.4). Work by the 'Nessos-painter', c. 620 BCE, National Archaeological Museum of Athens

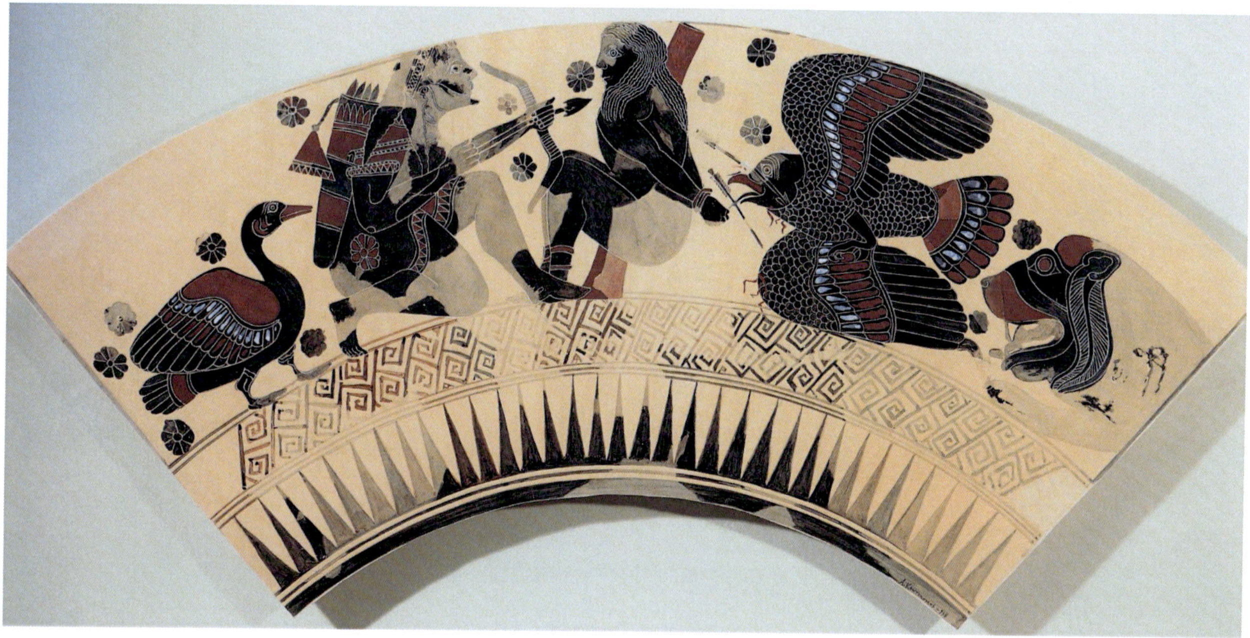

metheus in unbreakable, cruel chains and drove a pole through 'the middle'. Scholars nowadays, but as evidenced by the two objects, also artists back in the day weren't in consensus about what exactly was meant by the 'middle'. Was the pole driven through the middle of Prometheus, effectively impaling him? That seems to be the approach taken by the painter of the Attic krater. A different reading might be that the pole was driven through the middle of the chains behind Prometheus' back, like a column, as demonstrated by the artist who painted the Vatican bowl.

Fig. 2.4 Reconstruction of the painting on the Attic Skyphos krater from Athens, shown in Fig. 2.3 (From: Sofia Suli, Grecheskaya mifologiya, Athens, (Mihalis Tubis A. E.), 1995, p. 17)

AESCHYLUS' ROCKY PRECIPICE

For a very long time the Attic prototype, based on Hesiodos' telling – featuring Prometheus, the eagle, the column, and often, Herakles – is the sole type of illustration of the myth that can be found. This all changes in the fifth century BCE when a new author takes a crack

Fig. 2.5 On this relief from Aphrodisias we see Prometheus, with his arms spread, chained to a rocky precipice. The eagle lies slain by his side and Herakles is freeing Prometheus of his chains. In the background we see a nymph holding a throwing stick that she is throwing at the eagle, c. 150 BCE, Sebasteion temple complex, Aphrodisias (Turkey)

at retelling the myth: Aeschylus (c. 525-c. 456 BCE). This Athenian poet and playwright based a series of plays on the myth. The most well-known of these was a tragedy in three parts: *Prometheus bound, Prometheus unbound* and *Prometheus the fire-bringer*. Out of these three, only *Prometheus bound* has survived. One of the most profound differences between Aeschylus' and Hesiodos' handling of the myth is the moral judgement that befalls Prometheus. In Hesiodos' work Prometheus is an ambiguous figure, but in Aeschylus' telling, the Titan is transformed into a tragic hero, punished unjustifiably for his gift to humanity.

Aeschylus was part of the Athenian elite and wrote with an Athenian audience in mind. The city of Athens venerated Prometheus, with yearly torch processions celebrating the Titan as one of the protectors of city, together with the goddess Athena and the god Hephaistus. The common denominator between the three seems to be their association with knowledge, intelligence and crafts. All of these elements might explain why Prometheus was given a hero's role in the play by Aeschylus.

The influence of Aeschylus' tragedy was immediately visible in the depictions of the myth in visual arts produced in the fifth century BCE. One such work that exemplifies this development is a relief in the Sebasteion, a temple in Aphrodisias, Turkey (fig. 2.5). Prometheus' depiction has radically changed when compared to the art discussed earlier in this chapter: instead of being bound by his hands and feet and in a kneeling position, the Titan is chained to the rock (as opposed to the earlier column) with his arms outstretched in a way that evokes in a modern audience an association with a crucifixion. A possible theory that has been suggested by Olga Raggio for this exchange of column for rock comes from theatrical adaptation. Because Prometheus was a Titan, the offspring of primordial gods, the Titan as stage character would have needed to appear larger in stature than the other actors. This effect could be achieved by building a large, artificial Prometheus controlled by an actor concealed in the rock formation, operating the representation of the giant through handlebars and speaking through a theatrical mask.

Another new element introduced by Aeschylus that can be found in the Sebasteion relief is that Herakles frees Prometheus from his chains. The text by Hesiodos only men-

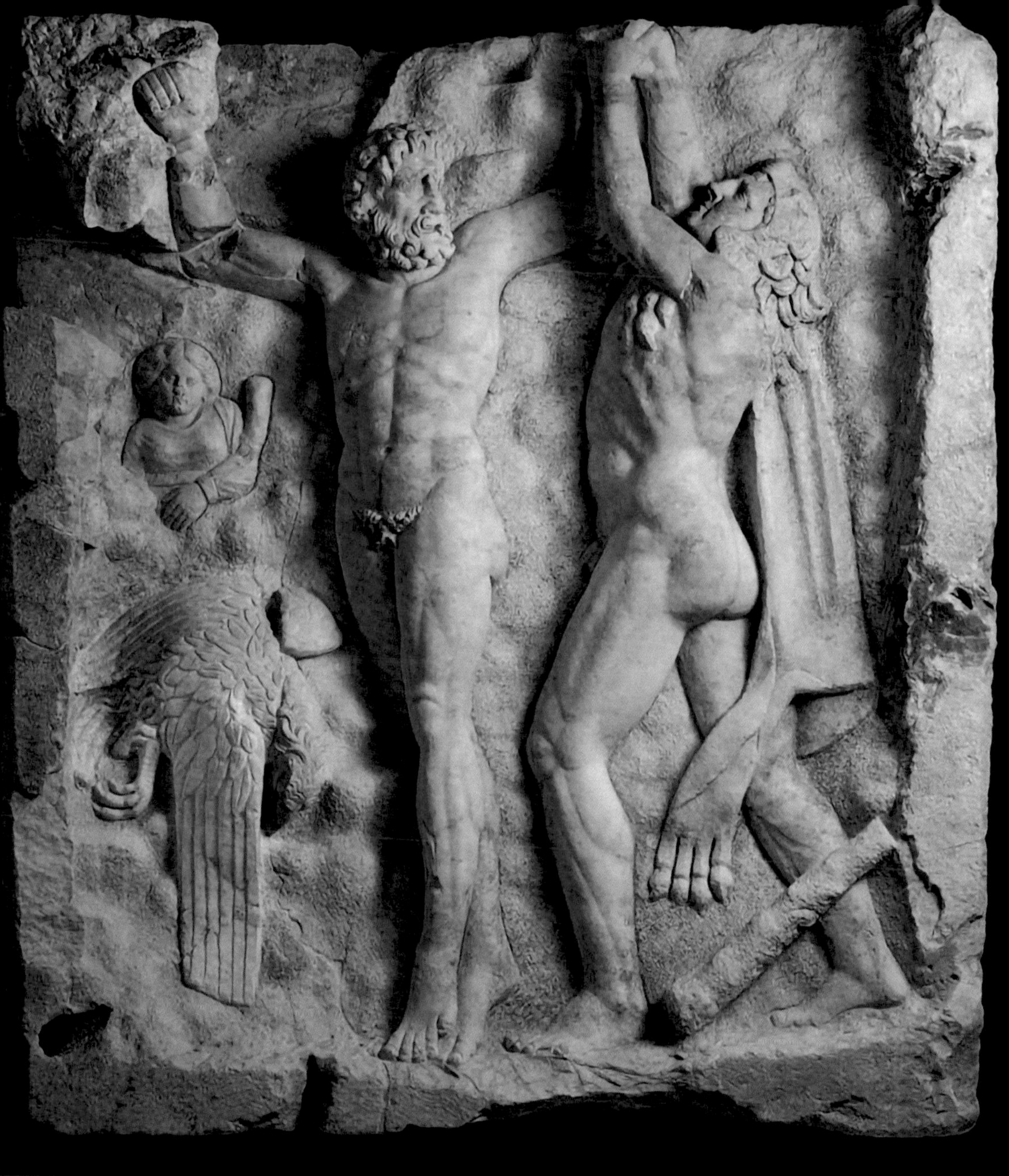

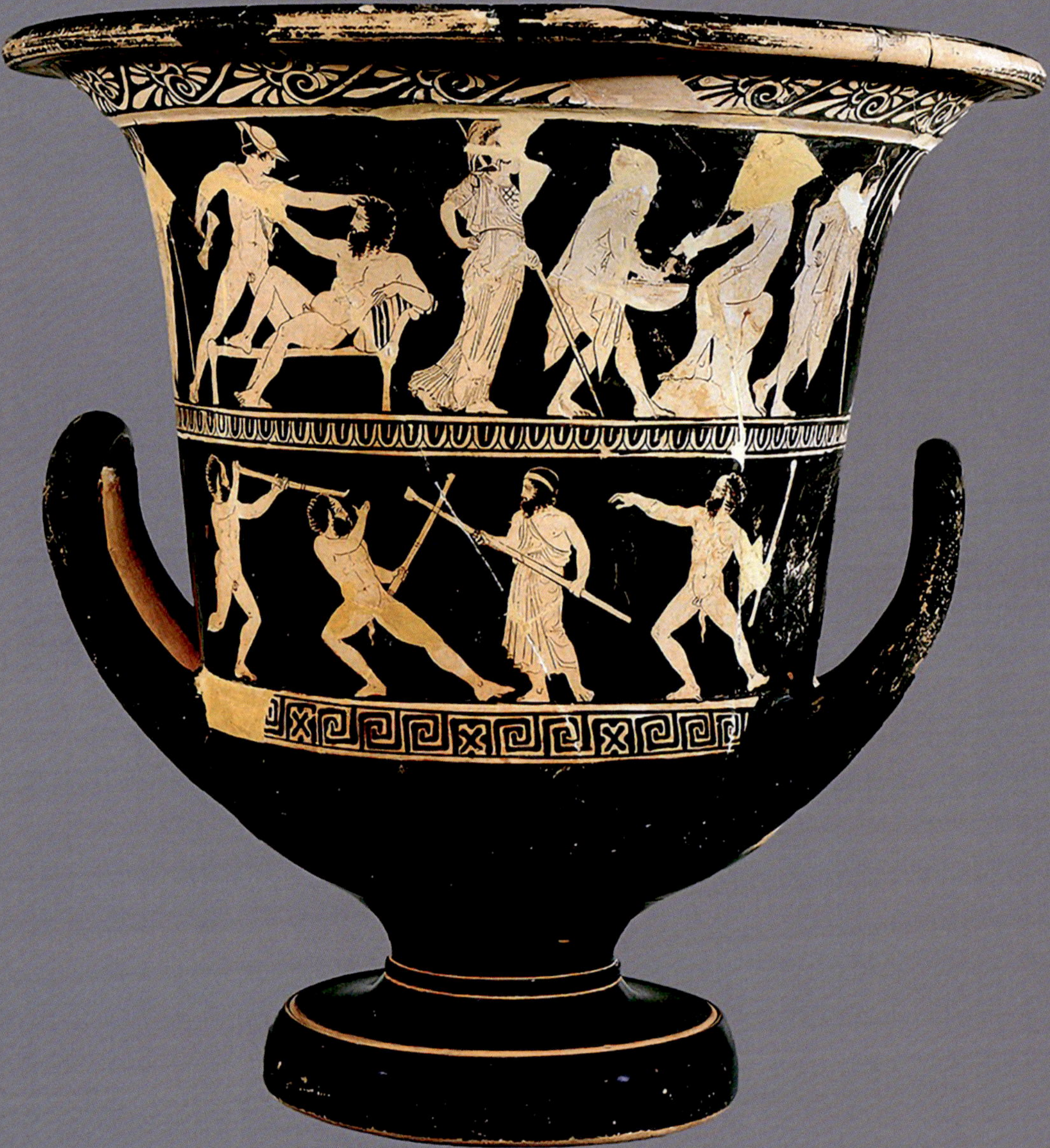

tions that Herakles kills the eagle, ending Prometheus' torment, but not necessarily freeing the chained Titan. Through mentions by other authors, we know that Herakles' freeing of the Titan was the topic of the second and now lost play by Aeschylus: *Prometheus unbound*. The relief at the Sebasteion is probably based on that play.

PROMETHEUS, BENEFACTOR OF THE SATYRS

We have knowledge of objects that seem to refer to other lost poetic works by Aeschylus. In addition to the Prometheus trilogy, he wrote a set of four satyr plays: short, tragicomical pieces where the choir consists of satyrs. They were themed around mythology but were rife with sexual innuendo, feigned drunkenness, and slapstick humour. To participate in literary competitions, Athenian playwrights always had to submit three tragedies and one satyr play, which would be performed either after the three tragedies or as an intermezzo between the third and second tragedy. This was to lighten up the heavy subject matter and long duration of the tragedies, and make it easier for the audience to endure them. The last of the four satyr plays is *Prometheus the fire-lighter*—some scholars have proposed that this satyr play and the last part of the trilogy *Prometheus the fire-bringer* are one and the same. Not much more is known about the contents of the play other than that Prometheus brings the fire to the first mortals, who, in this telling, aren't the humans but rather satyrs. Although this text has not survived, we can still identify references to it in Greek vase painting. An example of this is a red-figured Athenian krater held in the Ashmolean museum in Oxford (fig. 2.6). The subjects of the vase were historically misidentified as relating to Dionysus, the god of wine and revelry. Looking closely, however, one can see the name "Prometheus" painted alongside the central figure. The vase is divided vertically in two bands to narrate separate stories of Athenian heroes. In the upper band, we see several episodes of the life of Theseus. In the lower band, we see Prometheus (third from the left) accompanied by several satyrs. Prometheus appears calm and dignified, in stark comparison to the wild, rambunctious movements of the naked satyrs – identified in kind with painted names as Simos, Komos and Sikinnis –

Fig. 2.6 Red figure Athenian vase, the upper band shows scenes the heroic works of Theseus. The lower band shows Prometheus and three satyrs, identified as Sikinnis, Komos, and Simos. Prometheus holds the fennel stalk that he used to bring the fire; the satyrs are using it to light their torches, c. 425 BCE, Ashmolean Museum, Oxford

Fig. 2.7 Etruscan bronze mirror. Prometheus is freed from his chains. All figures are identifiable through inscriptions on the edge of the mirror. From left to right this reads Esplace (Aesclepius), Promanthe (Prometheus), Menrva (Minerva/Athena) and Hercle (Hercules/Herakles). Aesclepius, the god of medicine, binds the wound Prometheus' right side, Hellenistic, early 3rd century BCE, h. 27,9 cm, diam. 14,5 cm. Metropolitan Museum, New York City

who dance around the Titan. These are archetypical satyr names found across multiple satyr-plays by a wide variety of authors. Prometheus is holding his fennel stalk – the so-called *Narthex,* a species of giant fennel native to Greece – in his hand. This is the fennel stalk that, according to myth, he used to carry the fire down from Mount Olympus. The fennel stalk clearly differs from the torches carried by the satyrs, who are holding torches made out of bundles of pine twigs bound together, in Classical fashion.

The stories depicted on this vase refer to myths that held special significance for the city of Athens. It has been mentioned previously that part of the veneration of Prometheus in Athens included a torch procession and large, theatrical contests often preceding religious festivals. It is very possible that the end of the play *Prometheus the fire-lighter* transitioned into such a procession with "Prometheus" at the front, followed by the satyrs and finally the audience, all carrying lit torches. The vase in that case could give,a glimpse into what such a procession might have looked like.

PROMETHEUS WITH THE ETRUSCANS

For each of the artworks we've studied thus far, a literary source has inspired the manner the Promethean myth is depicted, even when the original text has been lost. There are, however, myriad objects that depict parts of 'Prometheus stories' within unknown literary sources. Surprisingly, several of these depictions are found in Etruscan sites on the Italian peninsula—not in Greece – where one might expect to find such objects. This is likely due to the rigorous trading network between these ancient Italian peoples and ancient Greece. The Etruscans also had a real fondness for Greek art; more Greek painted vases have been found in Etruscan tombs than in Greece itself. Additionally, Etruscan script was also based on Greek script, and the Greek gods were adopted into their own Italian pantheon. With the Etruscans, we find depictions of Prometheus that don't have comparable types in Greece, demonstrating the intermingling of the ancient Greek myth with a new, distinctly Italian narrative. Examples of this hybridity can be found in two bronze mirrors.

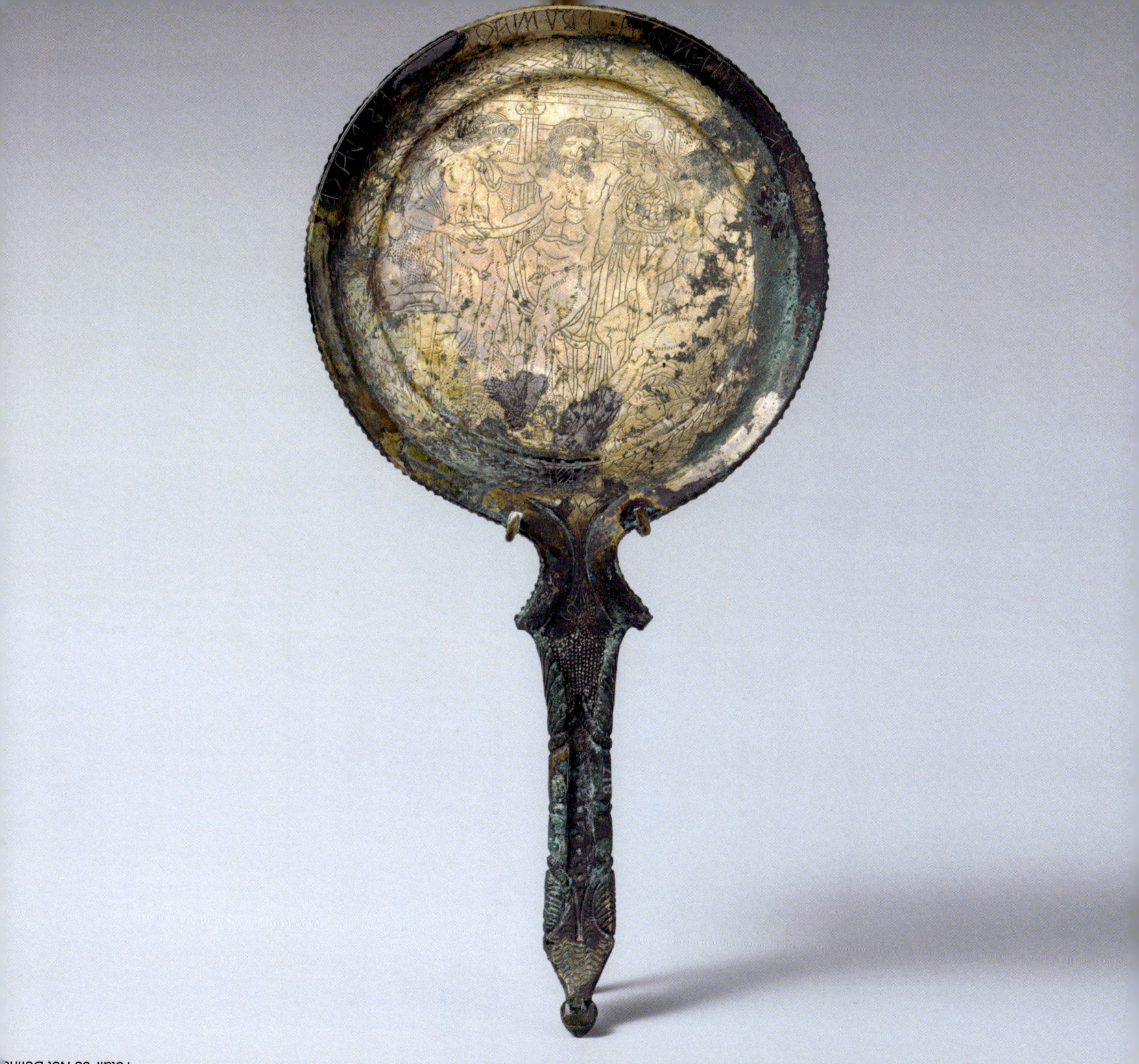

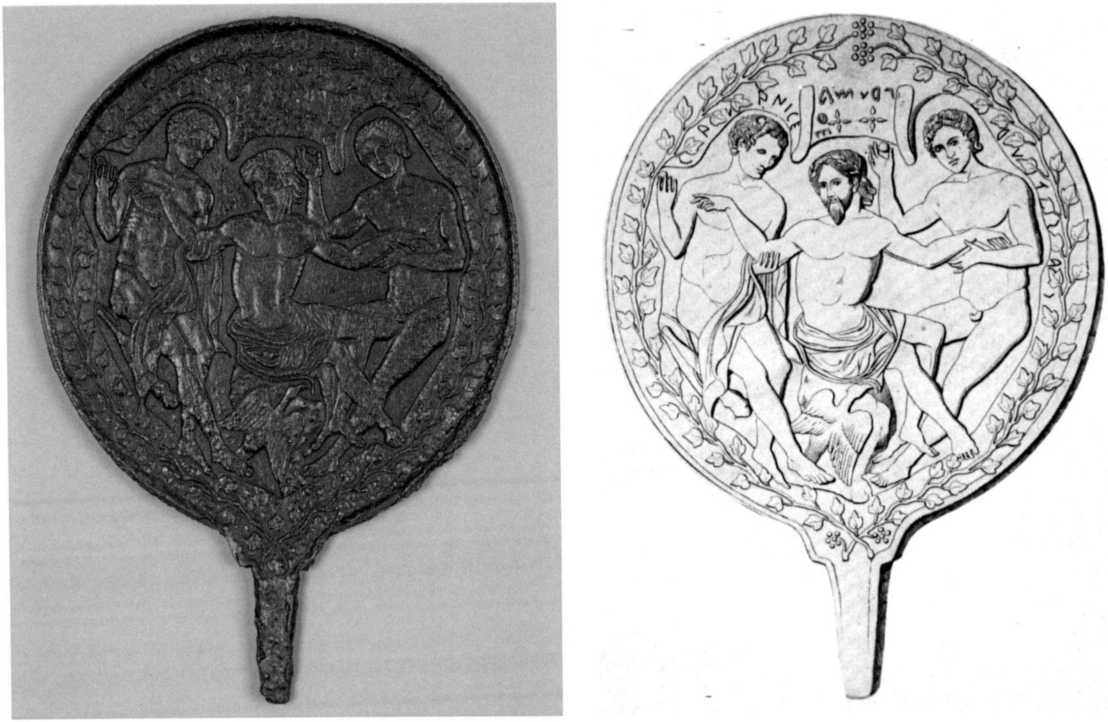

Fig. 2.8 The return of Prometheus on Olympus. The figures are identified by names written above their heads or on a text scroll above the central figure. In the center we find 'Prumethe', the etruscan spelling of Prometheus, with two flowers. The figure to the left is referred to as 'Kalanike' (Herakles Kallanikos, the divinised Herakles) and to the right we find 'Kastur' (Castor). Prometheus is carried heavenward by an eagle. Etruscan bronze mirror: Object (a) and reconstruction (b), discovered near Vulci in what used to be Etruria, c. 460-440 BCE, 17 x 23,5 cm, National Museum in Krakow

The first mirror, currently in the Metropolitan Museum of Art in New York City, contains a scene that could possibly stem from Aeschylus' tragedy *Prometheus unbound* (fig. 2.7). The way the scene is depicted, however, is completely unlike earlier illustrations, such as the relief from Aphrodisias (fig. 2.5). The unchained Prometheus is leaning – like the wounded Christ during the deposition from the cross – on the shoulders of Athena at his left; at his right, Asclepius, the god of medicine, treats the wound in his side and bandages him. All figures can be identified by inscriptions of their Etruscan names found on the edge of the mirror. From left to right we find the names: 'Esplace'(Asclepius), 'Prumanthe' (Prometheus), 'Menrva' (Minerva/Athena) and 'Hercle' (Hercules/Herakles). In contrast with earlier depictions, Herakles is not occupied in the act of saving Prometheus, as he has completed his task – the slaying of the eagle. The bird lies dead beneath the feet of Prometheus. The hero has stripped off his lion's pelt, which he sits on, at rest after completing his task.

The presence of Athena and Asclepius is new; the two are not typically seen in depictions of the liberation of Prometheus. The connection between Athena and Prometheus seems to be constituted by their bonds with the city-state of Athens, where they were venerated together as patrons of wisdom and technical knowledge. This could explain her presence in this scene. The role of Asclepius is perhaps more practical: as the god of medicine, he is needed for his expertise. With gentle care, he wraps a bandage around Prometheus' waist to dress the wound caused by the years of torment by the eagle.

At the back of the mirror—typically the reflective side—the word 'suthina' is carved in large letters. The term means 'for the grave'. Mirrors like this one were given by the Etruscans as grave gifts. In order to ensure that they wouldn't be stolen from the tombs, they rendered the mirrors useless for the living: they were no longer reflective. To achieve this, the Etruscans scratched on the reflective side so that the beholder could no longer look upon their own visage.

In the second mirror, c. 460-440 BCE held in National Museum in Krakow, we see Prometheus depicted as a suffering god (fig. 2.8). Once again, he's flanked by two figures.

This type of composition is frequently present on Etruscan mirrors. The scene depicted on this second mirror, however, is different from the previous mirror. Here, we see the return of Prometheus to Olympus. Once again, inscriptions identify the figures. In a large scroll above his head, Prometheus is once again signified as 'Prumanthe'. The figure to his left is identified as 'Kalanike', an Etruscan spelling referring to an epithet of the divine Herakles, – since Herakles was deified after his death – or 'Herakles Kallinikos,' which means 'beautiful victor'.

The other figure is identified as 'Kastur' or Castor, one half of the mythological heroic twins Castor and Pollux, the so-called Dioscuri. These sons of Zeus and Leda were very important deities to the Etruscans and they passed their veneration on to the Romans. The twins were legendary warriors that came back to life to lead the army whenever they were needed. To the Etruscans, however, they also filled another role: they could be called upon as guides of the soul on the final journey to the afterlife. Because they themselves had returned from the dead again and again, they were able to move between death and immortality. Below Prometheus' feet, we can see an eagle. It might be tempting to read this as the bird slain by Herakles, but this eagle is alive and charged with carrying Prometheus to skyward. This is an apotheosis, a motif seen in ancient Roman art in which the souls of the deified dead are carried into the afterlife by an eagle. The presence of the two companions, one a guide of souls into the afterlife, and the other a version of the deified Herakles, strengthens the assumption that this is image shows the apotheosis of Prometheus. It is the ultimate triumph for Prometheus: he has survived his torment and imprisonment and is now carried back to Olympus in the talons of the very bird who served as his torturer.

PROMETHEUS, CREATOR OF MANKIND

We have yet to examine one central part of the myth of Prometheus: Prometheus as creator of mankind. This absence is due to the fact that Prometheus is, in neither the texts of Hesiodos nor Aeschylus, not responsible for the creation of men. In these stories, this

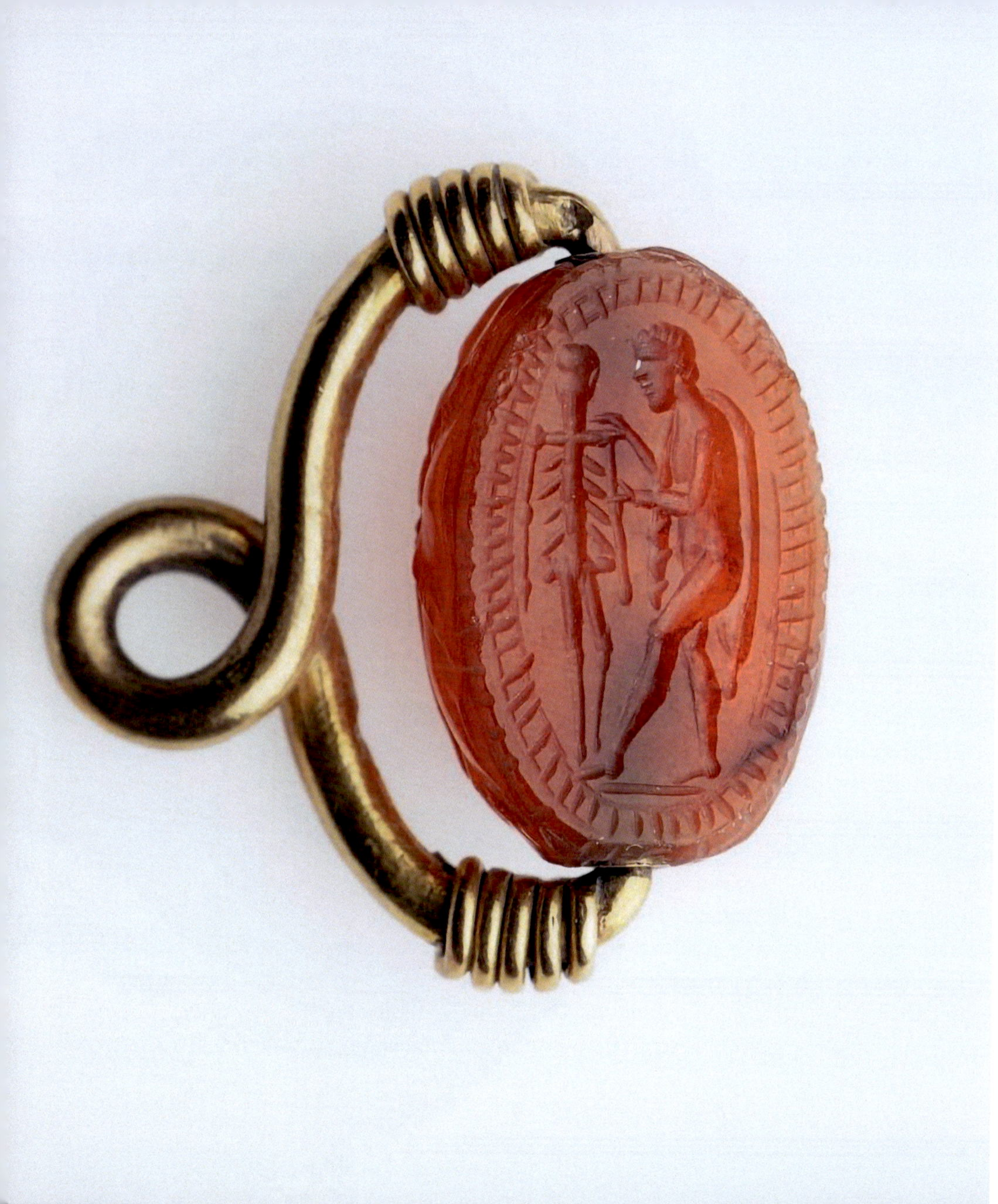

Fig. 2.9 Prometheus creates humans, the unfinished human is depicted as a skeleton. Roman engraved gemstone of the 'Scarab-type', intended as pendant for a necklace, carnelian, diam. 14 mm, ca. 100 BCE, Museum of Fine Arts, Boston

act was either completed by other gods, or the existence of humans was not explained. Prometheus is solely mankind's benevolent benefactor, giving them fire and the ability to cultivate knowledge. We begin to see references to Prometheus as the creator of men in ancient Greece around the fourth century BCE. The comedians Philemon and Menander make small references to this in works on different topics. However, there are no literary or artistic sources that would indicate that this part of the myth was widespread or popular.

The popularity of this role was completely different outside the Hellenistic world. Throughout the Roman Empire, the myth of Prometheus as creator of humans was incredibly popular. Ovid begins the Prometheus story in the *Metamorphoses* by relating how the Titan created humans. This theme can also be found in Roman art: especially in engraved gems, such as a gem now in the Boston Museum of Fine Arts (fig. 2.9). Engraved gems of this kind were called 'scarabs' because the rounded, intact side was modelled after the shield shape of the scarab beetle. These stones could be hung from necklaces as pendants. On this piece we see Prometheus using a chisel to create the first human, which is shown as a skeleton, held in an unfinished state.

In this chapter, we have seen how the Prometheus myth developed in ancient Greece and was taken on and transformed by various authors. These evolving, new versions of the story were taken up by artists of the age. The myth spread far outside of Greece, leading to the development of diverse regional variations unbeknownst to the Greek originators of the myth. The Romans added the new and influential detail of Prometheus as the creator of mankind – a part of the story that took on a life of its own in the onset of the Middle Ages, as will be expanded upon in the sixth chapter.

In the play by Aeschylus, Prometheus developed as the protector of the skilful human. The lessons that Prometheus gave mankind are not limited to skills that require the use of fire, like blacksmithing and baking clay. Aeschylus writes Prometheus a monologue in which the Titan lists all he has taught humanity, including, among other lessons: wearing rings, medicine, astronomy, and divination (reading the entrails of animals). Prometheus wasn't called 'he who looks ahead' for nothing. He gave mankind all the skills that required creative insight and a long-term vision. In the world of medicine, both of these traits have proven essential in the treatment of patients and development of the discipline.

But how far did the knowledge of the ancient Greeks on the properties of the liver extend? Prometheus' torment—in which his liver regrows nightly—suggests that they were at least aware that a liver is needed to sustain even an immortal life. In the ancient world, knowledge on the anatomical properties of the liver was rudimentary and mostly based on observations of the livers of animals. The next chapter shall expand on all these subjects with special attention for an Etruscan bronze model of a sheep's liver. We shall see the role the liver was given by the ancient Greeks and Etruscans and how it was used in divination practice.

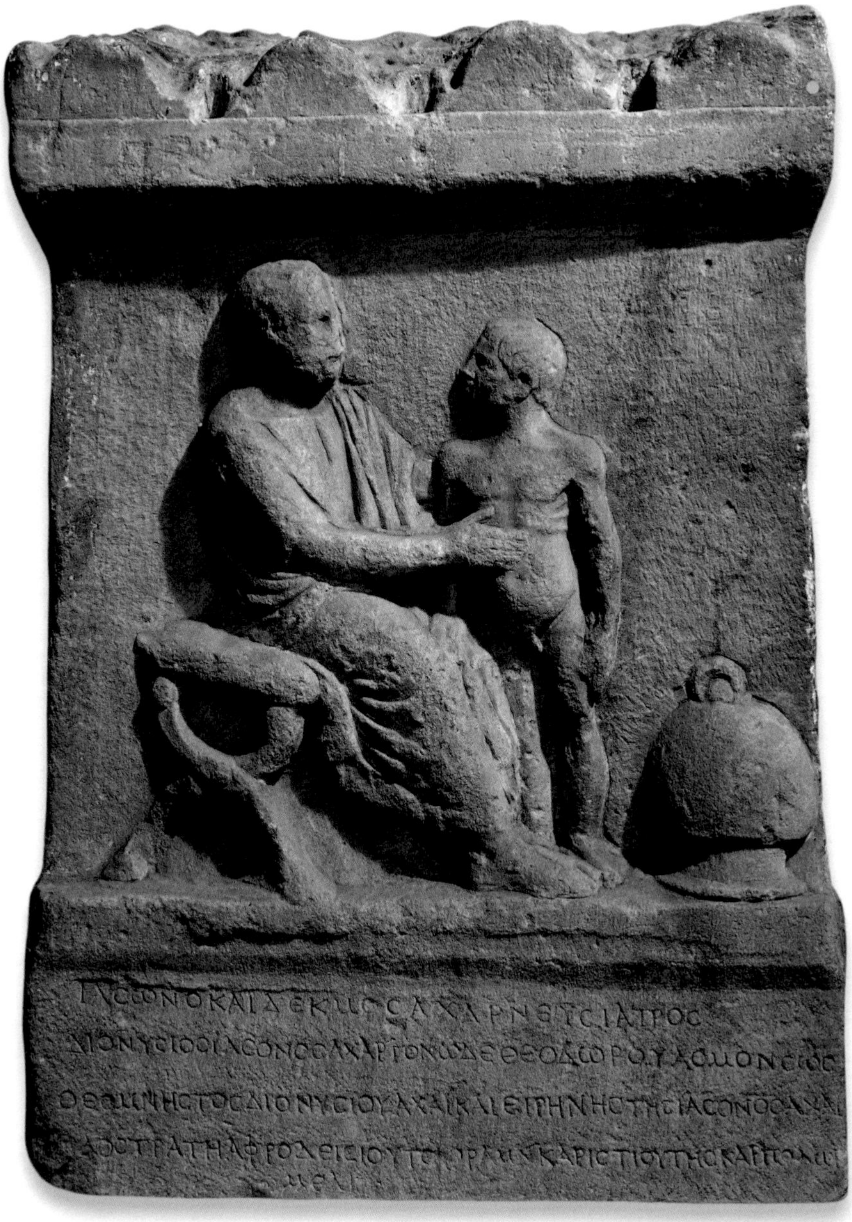

3

THE LIVER ACCORDING TO THE ANCIENT GREEKS AND THE ETRUSCANS

Ancient Greek medicine achieved its zenith in the figure of Hippocrates (ca. 460-377 BC). This physician, native to the isle of Kos, is seen as the father of Western medicine (fig. 3.1). The Hippocratic Oath, the foundational pledge of medical ethics that binds physicians to the ethical and standardized care of their patient, is still pledged by newly inaugurated doctors worldwide. Rational thoughts, based on Hippocrates' own observations and experiences, formed the cornerstone of his medical manifesto. He operated on the basis of humoral pathology in which four temperaments were distinguished and coupled to four types of bodily fluids: blood, phlegm, black gall and white gall. If a

Afb 3.0 The Greek physician Jason palpates a patient's liver in the upper abdomen. Ancient Greek gravestone, 2nd century BCE, British Museum, London

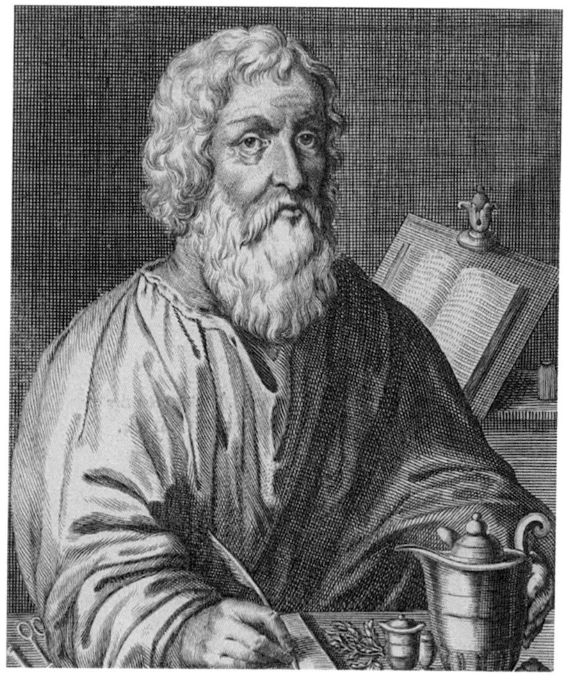

Fig. 3.1 Portrait of Hippocrates of Kos, by Pieter Philippe, 1635-1702, engraving, 167 x 103 mm, Rijksmuseum, Amsterdam

person fell ill, it indicated an imbalance of the humours, and the task of medicine was to restore this disrupted balance through, most commonly, a change in diet and lifestyle. Hippocrates' anatomical knowledge was sparse, and limited to what he could observe in the dissection of animals.

THE LIVER IN HIPPOCRATIC MEDICINE

According to Hippocrates, the liver was the dominant organ on the right side of the body, and the spleen occupied the left side. The liver was characterised by five lobes with the gallbladder attached to the fourth lobe. The 'mouth' of the gallbladder was directed towards the diaphragm, the lungs and the heart. The portal vein isn't described as such. Hippocrates discusses two main veins. One was supposed to spring forth from the liver and nourish the right half of the body, branching off towards the brain. The other was supposed to emerge from the spleen and nourish the left side of the body and a small-

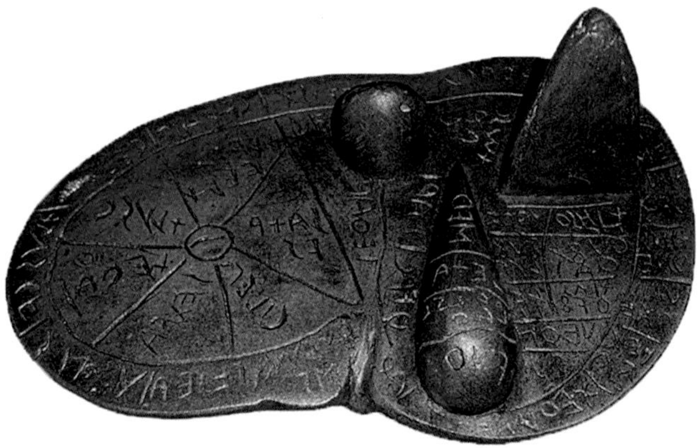

Fig. 3.2 Etruscan bronze model of a sheep's liver that was discovered near Piacenza, soothsayers used these types of models to predict the future, c. 100 BCE, 7,5 x 12,5 cm, Musei Civici di Palazzo Farnese, Piacenza

er part of the brain. These descriptions of the gallbladder and the major blood vessels around the liver indicate that knowledge of the anatomical features of the liver was still rudimentary in Hippocratic medicine. Hippocrates got one thing right: bile was formed in the liver and the build-up of this substance and subsequent congestion within the liver caused jaundice, the yellowing of skin and eyes.

THE BRONZE LIVER OF PIACENZA

In the small town of Piacenza, not far from Milan, we find the Palazzo Farnese. In 1550, this was the noble palace of the duke of Parma; today, it houses an archaeological museum with a very special Etruscan model of a sheep's liver cast in bronze (fig. 3.2). The Etruscans were an ancient people with a unique language, religion and culture. In a period spanning one thousand years – between ca. 1000 and 30 BCE – they lived in an area that today makes up the modern Italian regions of Tuscany, Latium and Umbria. The Etruscans were a highly advanced people; central to their societies were a polytheistic religion and ritual. One such ritual included divination. Etruscan oracles could 'read' the livers of sheep, that is to say predict the future based on the shape and position of the liver lobes – an art called 'hepatoscopy'.

The bronze liver at the Palazzo Farnese was found in 1877 in a field near Piacenza. The model is around 7.5 to 12.5 cm and is roughly dated to the year 100 BCE. It shows the lower side (the visceral side) of a sheep's liver. This side represented the image that the Etruscans had of the universe: a microcosm that reflected the heavenly macrocosm. Moving through that macrocosm was a vast pantheon of gods to whom the Etruscans entrusted the course of the future, a trust built on a vision revealed through hepatoscopy. The lower side of the liver was divided by lines into quadrants, which were, in turn, divided into four additional regions (fig. 3.3). The regions corresponded with the dominions of the gods in the universe. In order to make clear which regions corresponded to which gods, their names were engraved in the bronze model. For example, the gallbladder is inscribed with the name of Neptune, the water god, to whom this reservoir of watery

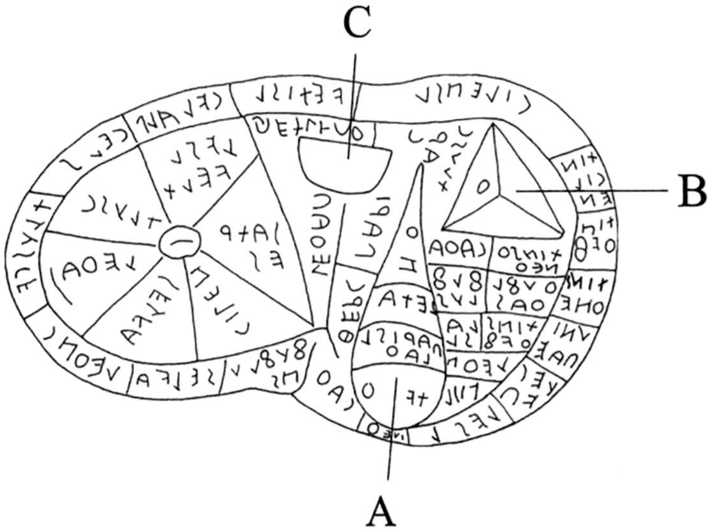

Fig. 3.3 Lower side of the bronze liver of Piacenza, divided in regions with inscriptions with the names of the Etruscan gods. Along the edge the bronze model is divided in 16 smaller regions that correspond with the gods in the central regions A) Galbladder, B) processus pyramidalis, C) processus papillaris

bile was dedicated. In a band around the bronze liver, we find sixteen smaller regions that were connected to the gods in the central regions. In this way, the Etruscans, dedicated to their faith as they were, assigned each god a place on their map of the universe, projected onto a sheep's liver.

The Etruscan model of the sheep's liver showcases several characteristic anatomical structures (fig. 3.2 and fig 3.3). The pear-shaped structure positioned at the centre of the model is the gallbladder (A), which is visible in its full length in a human or animal liver if the organ is lifted. The convex part of the gallbladder in those cases would be at the front and upper side of the liver. In the Etruscan model, however, the liver is reversed, with the convex part of the gallbladder pointing down—this is if one uses the inscribed letters as an orientation guide or instruction on how to hold the model. On the right side of the gallbladder, we find a pyramid-shaped structure that was referred to as the *processus pyramidalis* (B). This structure anatomically corresponds with the *caudate lobe* in humans, a small lobe on the backside of the liver with a spur that reaches into the (anatomical) right liver lobe. On the other side of the gallbladder, the bronze liver shows a protrusion shaped like a semi-circle (C) that was called the *processus papillaris* and corresponds – in humans – with an anatomical spur of the *caudate lobe* next to the caval vein. These three elements can also be found on clay models of sheep livers found in Babylonian civilisations (fig. 3.4), fifteen hundred years earlier in the town of Mari in ancient Syria. These clay models were similarly used for telling the future. The *processus pyramidalis* is clearly visible in the Babylonian liver, this time as a prism shaped protrusion (a) to the left of the gallbladder (b).

Fig. 3.4 Babylonian clay model of a sheep's liver that was used for soothsaying, the processus pyramidalis is recognisable as a prism-shaped protrusion (b), to the left of the gallbladder (a). c. 2000 BCE, 7,5 x 6,9 cm, Musée du Louvre, Paris

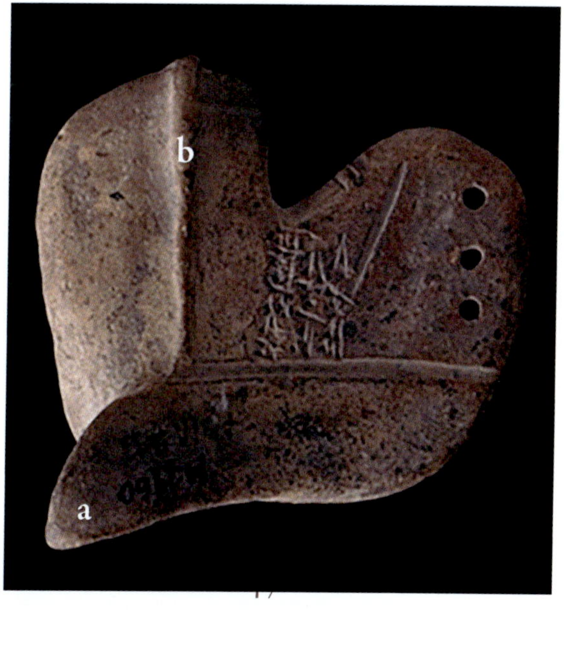

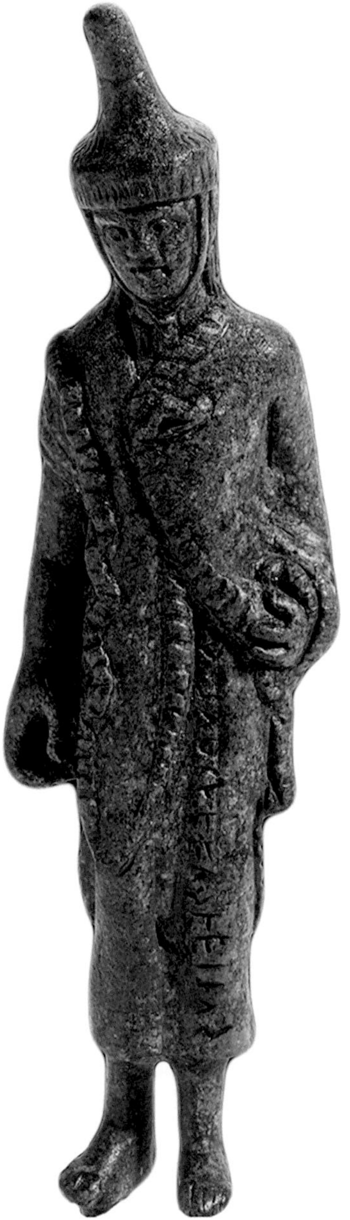

4

THE HARUSPEX AND HEPATOSCOPY

Within ancient Etruscan culture the *haruspex*, the oracle, fulfilled an important societal function. He (women were excluded from fulfilling this role) foretold the hidden intentions of the gods – and thus the future – by reading animal entrails. Most often the future was read in the liver of a sacrificed sheep. The aforementioned bronze liver found in Piacenza served as an instructive model for students who were training to become *haruspex* (fig. 3.2). The *haruspex* would cut the liver out of the sheep, hold it up in his left hand and run his right hand over the base of the organ. He would then inspect the liver clockwise. Figure 4.1 shows a statue of a *haruspex* on the lid of an urn, now in the Etruscan Museum of Volterra. The oracle is depicted practicing his craft, holding

Afb 4.0 Image of an Etruscan soothsayer, the haruspex, recognisable by his mantle and pointed cap that was fastened with a chinstrap. Bronze, 4th century BCE, Vatican Museum, Rome

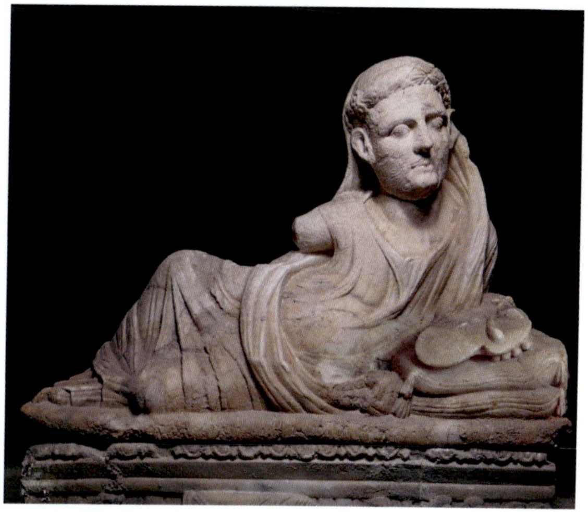

Fig. 4.1 Urn with on the lid a haruspex holding, in his left hand, a sheep's liver. He extends the underside to the spectator, causing them to see the liver upside down, with the round side of the gallbladder pointed downward, Etruscan Museum of Volterra, Museo Guarnacci

the liver in his left hand and showing the underside of the organ to the spectator. Beholders of this spectacle would view the liver upside down--the convex side of the gallbladder pointing downward instead of upwards (the position it occupies within the body). This presents one explanation for the upside down orientation of the bronze liver from Piacenza.

The protrusions on the lower side of the liver, the *processus pyramidalis* and the *processus papillaris*, formed two points of reference during 'hepatoscopy', the art of predicting the future based on the presence and shape of these protrusions. Pliny the Elder, the famed Roman encyclopaedist, described these two structures, writing that they could vary greatly in appearance. It is these variations in shape that formed the basis for reading the organ in divination. The *processus pyramidalis*, also called the *caput*, was the most significant structure in the construction of fortunes. If the *caput* was absent, this was seen as an ill omen. If either of the two protrusions appeared in duplicate however, this was seen as a good sign and a promise of prosperity. When important decisions had to be made, such as the beginning of a military campaign or starting a voyage, a liver reading would be consulted and the final decision thus placed in the hands of the gods.

Are the anatomical properties of a sheep's liver so striking that the future can be read in them? In order to study the variable shapes of the *processus pyramidalis* and *papillaris,* we examined ten fresh livers provided to us by an artisanal meat processing company. These livers belonged to adult sheep and were about the same weight as a human liver (ca. 1,5 kg). A lamb's liver weighs about 800 grams, a weight better suited to be held in one hand. Following in the footsteps of the *haruspex*, we held the livers up in our left hands and noted the attributes of the *processus pyramidalis* and *papillaris*.

We were struck by how varied both of these structures were among the ten livers: the *processus pyramidalis* consistently showed three triangular planes in each liver but greatly varied in size and length. The *processus papillaris* showed the most variation (fig. 4.2): it could be large, small, with or without ridges and, in one liver, it was absent altogether – a bad omen according to the Etruscans. This bad omen, however, was countered by two other livers where the *processus papillaris* presented in duplicate! It goes without saying that the *haruspex* was extremely skilled at recognising the anatomical varieties in sheep's livers. He had to be: the Etruscan future depended on his divinations.

The ancient Greeks clearly had little knowledge of the anatomy and function of the human liver. Yet, in Greek mythology, the liver was considered the seat of life in both gods and men. The liver was inferred religious and mystical properties; Etruscan oracles could 'read' the future in a sheep's liver. To have Prometheus' liver eaten away by an eagle, probably was the most severe punishment one could envisage at that time.

Fig. 4.2 Fresh sheep's liver where the galbladder (A) and the anatomical protrusions of the processus pyramidalis (B) and processus papillaris (C) are visible. The processus papillaris is small in this liver and only appears once.

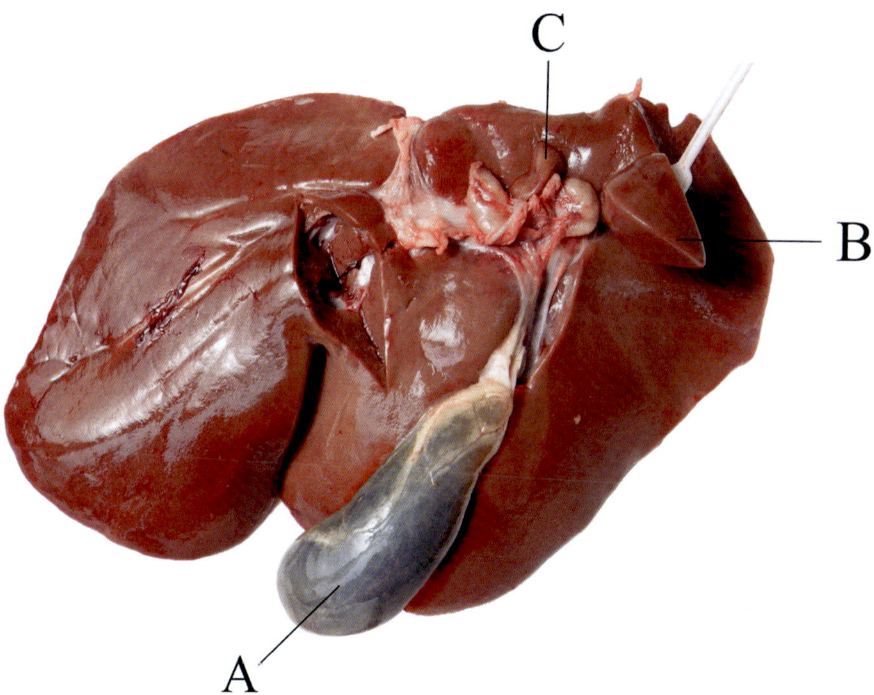

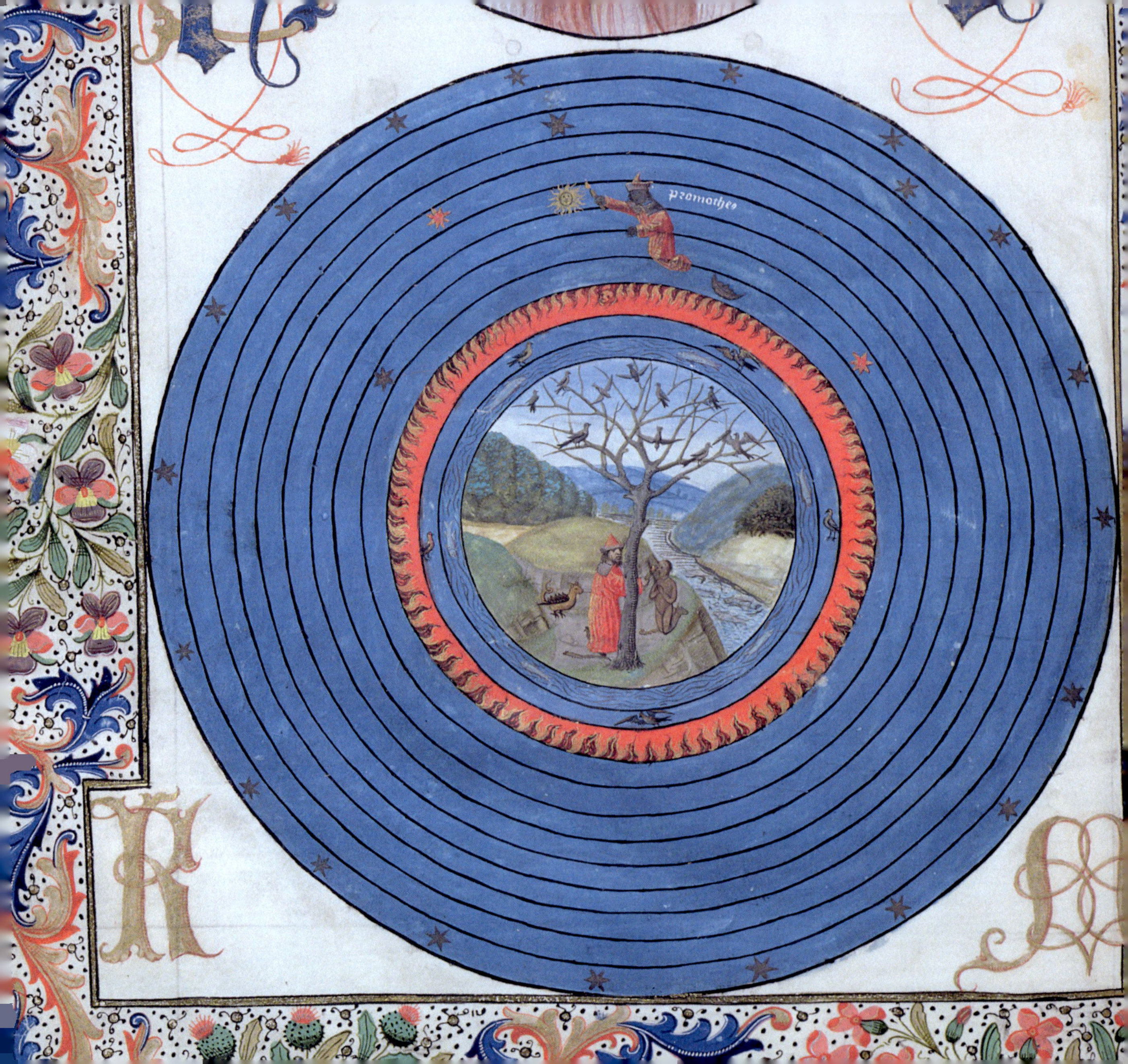
promotheꝰ

5

PROMETHEUS IN THE MIDDLE AGES

One of the most significant changes in the cultural landscape between antiquity and the Middle Ages is the rise and spread of Christianity in Europe. The new faith brought with it new stories that required new modes of depiction. This raises the question of what role a pagan classical figure like Prometheus could fulfil in this new world. In this chapter, we shall answer that question.

The Middle Ages are a time period that remains plagued by negative associations in the court of public opinion: It is seen as a dark period of decay, the remnants of the fall of the glorious ancient world, and a time where nothing noteworthy was produced in terms of art. It is not until the Renaissance that we would be relieved from this darkness. In reality, however, this characterisation is not justified. There are no hard lines between antiquity, the Middle Ages and the Renaissance. Rather, we ought to speak of a continuum: thoughts, stories, and images from antiquity did not vanish during the Middle Ages, and the seeds of Renaissance thought were already planted in the works of medieval scholars.

It's precisely because of this continuum that periodisation within art history is a point of contention amongst academics; defining a precise date range to correspond with a period is challenging if not impossible. In this chapter, we shall discuss a very long and thus

Fig. 5.0 We see the world, structured by a model using heavenly spheres. In the sphere belonging to the sun, Prometheus is stealing the heavenly fire. In the middle of the image, he uses the stolen fire to animate a human. Flemish, 15th century, 410 x 300 mm, Holkham, Holkham Hall, 324, fol. 13v

Fig. 5.1 Prometheus creates humans, mosaic, c. 218-238 CE, discovered in Edessa (Syria), private collection

pluriform period of nearly one thousand years, placed under the moniker 'the Middle Ages'. We shall follow depictions of Prometheus from the advent of Christianity to the fall of Constantinople in 1453.

Christian art can be first found in the later days of classical antiquity. Even when Christianity was not yet tolerated as a religion, and Christians were persecuted, Christian art was already produced in Rome. The same artisans that produced all other art, made works for Christian clients. When these artisans did this, they used the same models, style and figures as they would for pagan scenes, but by including certain elements or stories from Christian narrative, the images were given a Christian meaning.

CHRISTIAN STORIES, CLASSICAL IMAGERY

When it comes to Prometheus, the aforementioned intermingling of classical models and Christian stories can be located in a mosaic from the Syrian town of Edessa, dating from ca. 218 – 238 CE (fig. 5.1). This mosaic depicts the creation of man by Prometheus, accompanied by an assembly of Olympic gods. The figures are divided over two registers, splitting the picture vertically in two. In the lower register (reading from left to right), we see Hermes, recognisable by the two small wings on his head. He leads a young girl with butterfly wings to a stiff, standing figure in the front and centre of the composition. The winged, young girl is Psyche, the representation of the human soul. In classical mythology, Hermes guided the souls of the dead into the afterlife, and in this image, he fulfils this role as so called 'psychopomp' by guiding the human soul (Psyche) to the newly created human body that Prometheus has moulded out of clay. Also present is Amor, the lover and partner of Psyche depicted as a winged youth. In the mosaic, Amor encourages the hesitant soul to unify with the body. At the right of the composition, we see two additional lifeless clay figures, a man and a woman, propped against the frame of the picture.

In the upper register (this time read from right to left), the artist identifies certain figures with inscriptions. On the far right, we see a bearded man seated on a throne: this is Zeus, identified by his name in Syriac. The letters 'MRLH' to the right of his head mean

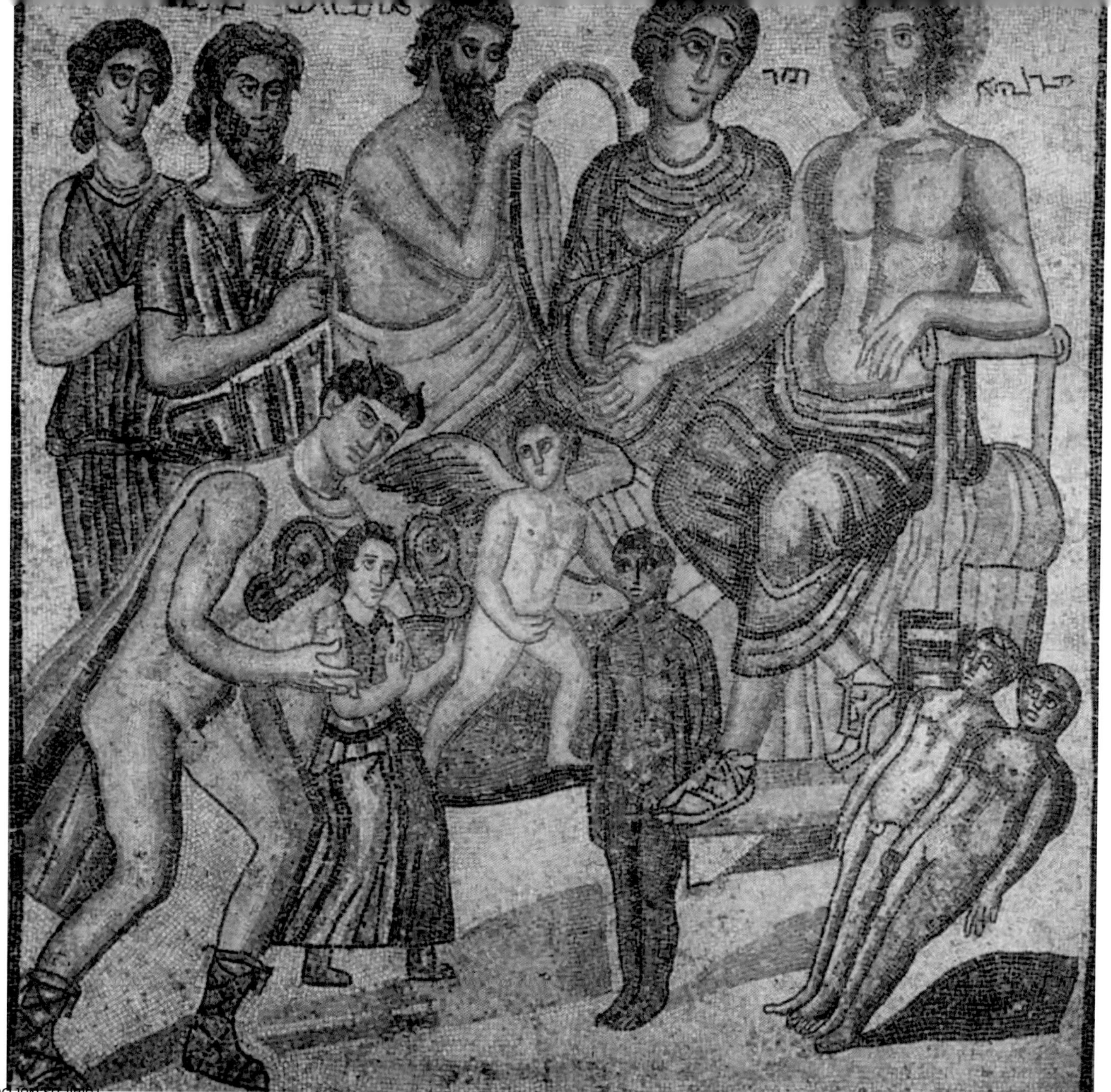

'Marallahe', which meant 'ruler of the gods'. Zeus is crowned with a nimbus as a sign of his divinity—this is one prevalent example of the transference of pagan iconography to Christian symbols. At the left, next to Zeus we find Hera, his spouse, who is identified with an inscription as well. The next figure in the row, an old man holding a hoop-shaped object in his hands, is not identified with an inscription, though the current consensus is that this figure is Aion, the god of time, who may be seen here holding the circle of the year with the seasons. To Aion's right is Prometheus, whose identity is proclaimed in the letters 'PRMTWS QRMWYS," written again in Syriac script and translated as 'Prometheus Kerameus', or 'Prometheus the ceramic.' This epithet refers to Prometheus' role as the 'sculptor' of mankind. The woman on the far left standing partially behind Prometheus is recognizable as the goddess Athena: patroness of ceramics and artisans. Due to her role as protector of artisans, she is often depicted accompanying Prometheus in his creation mythos. The goddess wears a *peplos*, a women's tunic bound together around the waist with a belt, one of her identifying attributes.

The myth of Prometheus as the creator of mankind gained greater popularity with the Romans than the Greeks. Syria in the third century CE was part of the larger Roman Empire, meaning that the popularity of this scene was not restricted to the Italian peninsula, but was indeed widespread through the entire empire. The scene on the mosaic is executed in a style that shows both Hellenistic influences (from the Graeco-Roman world) and near-Eastern influences. It's not just the subject matter that is classical: the balanced and harmonious composition, the suggestion of depth through the use of overlapping figures, and the use of naturalistic gradual shading are all Hellenistic stylistic characteristics. The eastern influence is best seen in the eyes of the figures: they all have large almond-shaped eyes with heavy eyelids that seem to look slightly upwards, as if the figures are lost in thought. The only figure that makes eye contact with one of the others is the clay human, who, instead of serenely staring into space, looks expectantly at his approaching soul (Psyche). Other eastern stylistic characteristics include the heavy outline on the figures, which gives the illusion that they are cut away from the background, and the uniformity of the silhouettes of the figures in the upper register. The artist may have been a local Syrian artisan who received a classical education.

The mosaic was made to decorate a grave in Edessa, a city that, at the time of the mosaic's production, was nearly exclusively Christian. This mosaic, as well as other mosaics with mythological subject, demonstrates that the Christian community did not eschew mythological imagery as long as that iconography could be read through a Christian lens. In the latter years of the Roman Empire during the transition towards the Middle Ages and the advent of Christianity, we often find Prometheus in funerary art. The fluid way in which certain pictorial models could be used in both pagan and classical readings becomes apparent when we place the mosaic in the context of other funerary art.

We want to make the comparison between the mosaic and a fourth-century painting found in the catacombs near the *Via Latina* in Rome (fig. 5.3). The patron that commissioned the grave chose an explicitly Christian scene. We see Christ as the most prominent figure in the foreground; he is dressed in white and beardless, portrayed in the act of resurrecting Lazarus from the dead. Lazarus' corpse, wrapped in a shroud, seems to stand stiffly in a small building, meant to signify a mausoleum. This theme of resurrection after death – the miracle performed by Christ in this New Testament story – was very fitting for a funerary image. The imagery used to depict this Christian message, however, was nearly identical to imagery used to depict pagan scenes, an outcome of the joint work that artisans who decorated the catacombs, the so called *fosors*, created for Christian and pagan clients alike. This overlap becomes especially apparent when we compare the image of Christ resurrecting Lazarus with an illumination one such pagan scene from a Roman manuscript dating from that same period (fig. 5.2). In this miniature, found within the the *Vergilius Vaticanus*—a richly illustrated manuscript dating from the early fifth century—we see a scene from the story of the demigod Aeneas. Queen Dido – at left – brings a sacrifice to

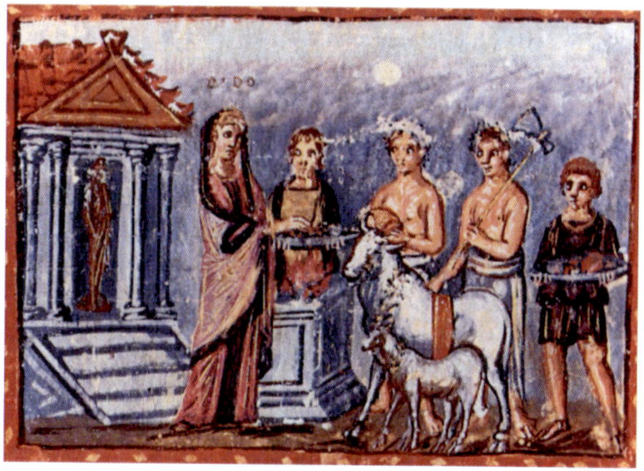

Fig. 5.2 Dido brings an offering, illustration from the Vergilius Vaticanus, c. 400 CE, h. 225 x w. 200 mm. Biblioteca Apostolica Vaticana, Rome, MS lat. 3225. fol. 33

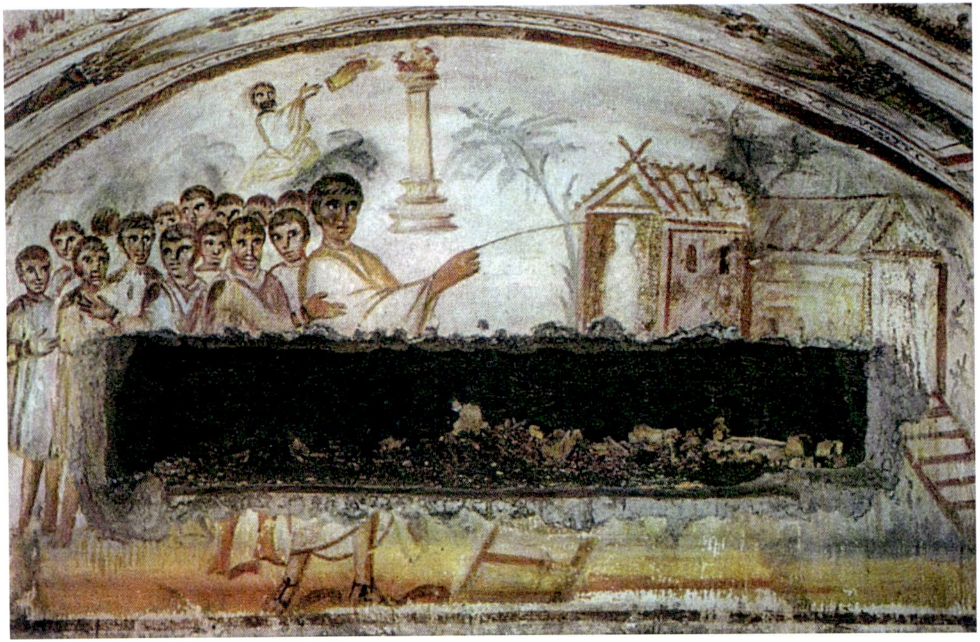

Fig. 5.3 The resurrection of Lazarus. Christ touches the head of the shrouded Lazarus, standing in a mausoleum, with his staff. Christ is accompanied by a large company of followers who all regard the miracle. The scene is damaged by a hole in the wall, this is the grave that contained the remains of the departed but that has since been opened, causing the plaster that once covered it to be peeled away. Fresco, 4th century CE, Catacomb by the Via Latina, Rome

the temple that can be seen behind her; through the gate of the temple, the beholder views a statue of the God who is receiving the sacrifice. There are definite similarities between the characteristics of the figures in both the Lazarus scene and the manuscript miniature, and this similarity is concretized in the near-identical mausoleum and the temple in Fig. 5.3. The pediment of both buildings shows two crossing beams, resulting in a 'V'-shape, and both buildings have stairs leading to their entrances. By wrapping the statue of the divinity in a shroud the classical topos has been cleverly adapted for a Christian context. We can extend this stylistic overlap to the Prometheus mosaic (fig. 5.1). The stiff and lifeless clay figures show great similarities to the lifeless body of Lazarus in his mausoleum, but also with the divinity in the temple. the statue, like them= figures, is a sculpture but according to roman faith such statues that still were 'embodied' by a divinity. Like the statue, the clay figures are inhabited by a soul, and like Lazarus, they are something lifeless brought to life. This connection goes beyond stylistic properties. Prometheus, like Christ, brought lifeless matter to life and animated it. In the catacomb the thematic connection is made between the body of the deceased and the resurrected Lazarus, in the mosaic the connection could be made between the body of the deceased and the clay figure brought to life. The union of soul and body, the animation of that which was previously lifeless, is a message that – when found on a grave – references the promise of resurrection during the end of days. This promise of resurrection was one of the central doctrines of early Christianity, and played a huge part in its appeal. It set the religion apart from the central Roman faith – worshipping the emperor and pantheon of the Olympic gods – and several other small so-called 'mystery cults' because it was the only religion that offered such a promise. The fact that the myth of Prometheus contained a narrative of unification between the soul and the body and relayed a story of the animation of lifeless matter made the myth suitable for Christian appropriation in stories of resurrection. It is because of these similarities that the myth could be used in a Christian funerary context.

We have now seen this narrative made subject in mosaics and wall paintings, but the due to its association with resurrection Prometheus' creation myth can also be found in a third type of funerary art: the sculpted reliefs on sarcophaguses. We will use two sarcophaguses to demonstrate that the link between the Prometheus myth and Christianity—and the fluidity between Christian and the art of antiquity—went beyond mere associations but one could serve as a model for the other. When we compare the Christian creation story, as told in Genesis, with the myth of Prometheus as creator, similar themes are instantly recognisable. In both narratives, humans are created out of earth or clay, which is then animated. Another strain that both stories share is a connection between the fall from grace and the introduction of knowledge to the world. Prometheus brought mankind knowledge by gifting them fire, but mankind was punished for this by means of Pandora who, when opening her chalice, brought evil to Earth and ended the paradisical state that humans had been living in up to that point. In the Christian story of creation, Eden is similarly ended by the introduction of knowledge, after the fruit of the tree of knowledge of good and evil is consumed.

PROMETHEUS: A 'GENESIS ACCORDING TO THE PAGANS'

The similarity between both Prometheus and God the Father creating out of clay, did not go unnoticed by early Christians. In the earliest centuries of Christianity, the creation of men in the myth of Prometheus was referred to as a *Genesis secundum gentiles*, which translates to 'genesis according to the pagans.' This connection between God the Father as creator and Prometheus is made explicitly in a relief carved into a third-century sarcophagus, now held at the Louvre (fig. 5.4). We see many compositional elements reminiscent of the aforementioned Edessa mosaic. A key difference between the Edessa mosaic and this sarcophagus relief is that Prometheus replaces Zeus, seated centrally on his throne, the clay human placed on a pillar before him (fig. 5.5). Once again Athena places a guiding hand on his shoulder and Psyche, the human soul, is guided towards the lifeless clay human by Hermes. The sarcophagus, however, depicts a more elaborate version of the cycle. The story is now supplemented with the inclusion of the 'Moirai', the

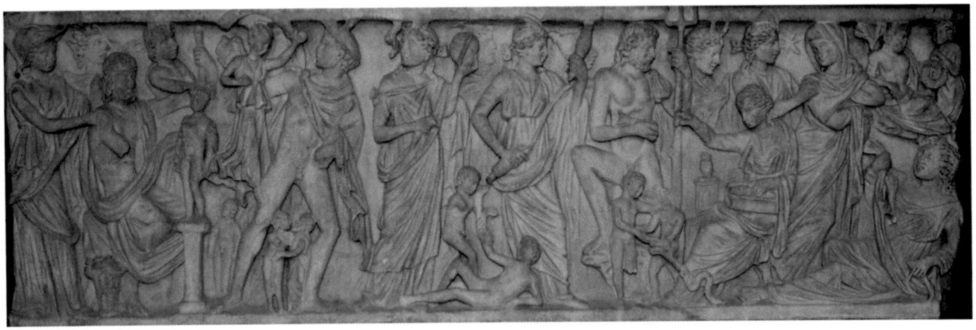

Fig. 5.4 Prometheus creates humans, relief on a Roman sarcophagus, 71 x 221 cm, Arles, c. 240 CE. Musée du Louvre, Paris

fates, who shape the life that will be lived by the first human. The first fate is constructing a horoscope for the human out of the rings of the zodiac; the second spins his life-thread which when cut spells the end of the human's life; and the last unfurls a scroll that relays the life of the human.

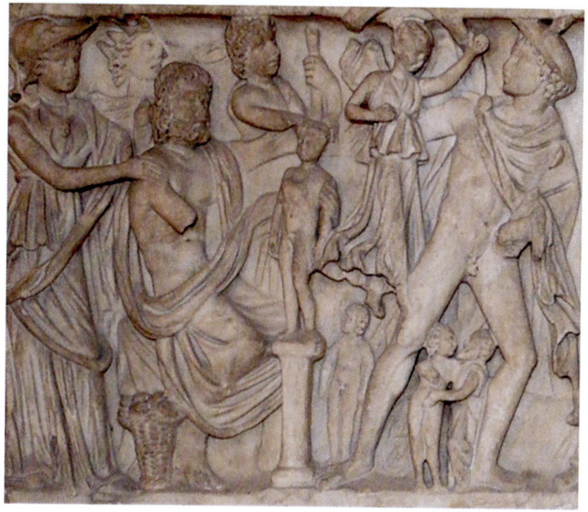

Fig. 5.5 Prometheus creates humans (detail of Fig. 5.4)

The Louvre sarcophagus was built and decorated in Arles in 240 CE to carry the remains of an unknown Roman, but its functionality did not end there. The sarcophagus was reused as the final resting place for Saint Hilary of Arles after his death in 449. This sanctified bishop was buried in a pagan sarcophagus! There is a dual explanation for this: on one hand, high-quality objects from antiquity were often reused in the Middle Ages due to their material and aesthetic value without much regard for the pagan origin. On the other,, the appropriateness of the Prometheus myth for Christian use may also have contributed to its use for a Christian Saint. Both the creation of mankind out of clay and the theme of resurrection reflect Christian principles. When a Saint dies, his or her corpse remains sacred and powerful. Objects that once belonged to the saint can be imbued with this sanctity, and this is especially true of the grave. This sarcophagus was regarded as such a relic. Pilgrims would travel far and wide to pray in front of it and to touch it, all the while hoping for a miracle.

Unfortunately, when the sarcophagus was transported to the Louvre, the lid—with Saint Hilary's name carved into it—remained in the archaeological museum of Arles (Musée de l'Arles et de la Provence antiques). Because of this separation, the sarcophagus that is exhibited at the department of classical art became divorced from its second life as a medieval object of great significance. A visitor that sees the sarcophagus today would only view it in its pagan and antique context and not as an object of great importance to medieval French Christianity. This separation denies the fact that the sarcophagus has played an important role in both pagan and Christian contexts.

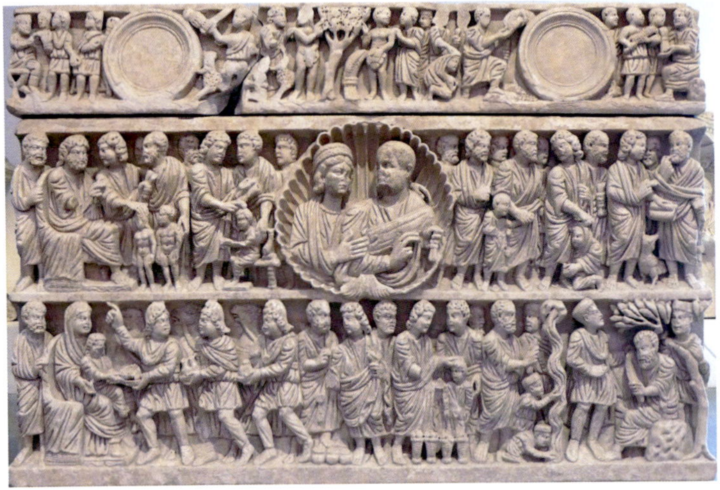

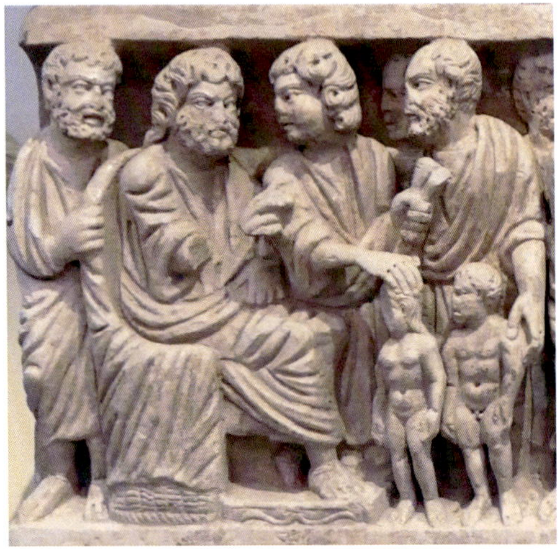

Fig. 5.6 Trinity sarcophagus, marble, c. 315 CE, Musée de l'Arles et de la Provence antiques, Arles

Fig. 5.7 Trinity sarcophagus (detail of Fig. 5.6)

The religious associations with Prometheus become explicit when we regard the emergence of a new pictorial model in Christian sarcophaguses. By means of comparison with these sarcophaguses it becomes apparent that the sarcophagus in the Louvre, as well as other Prometheus sarcophaguses of the same type, have directly influenced Christian art. This can be seen in the reliefs decorating the so called 'trinity sarcophagus,' also produced in Arles (fig. 5.6 and 5.7).

This sarcophagus was produced around the year 315 CE, about seventy years after the so-called Prometheus sarcophagus at the Louvre. It contains solely Christian imagery. In the upper left corner, the Christian creation of man is depicted. The sarcophagus tries to render one of the most complex dogmas of the Church in a visual form: that of the nature of the trinity, which simultaneously consisted of separate entities, but yet was one and the same. The theoretical, spiritual, and philosophical questions surrounding this dogma were the topic of fierce debate within the early Christian community and these debates produced schisms within the Church. This sarcophagus attempts to formulate a visual answer to the question of how to interpret the trinity by depicting the three aspects of the trinity as three separate figures that are simultaneously working together in the creation of humanity. God the Father is seated on a throne, The Holy Spirit is standing behind him with a hand on his shoulder and a young, beardless Christ has his hand on the head of Eve. The similarities in composition and subject between this sarcophagus and the Prometheus sarcophagus are evident. Prometheus, the creator, is seated on a throne, and Athena, here functioning as a personification of reason, fulfils a similarl spiritual role as the Holy Ghost, positioned behind the Titan. Finally, Hermes, who guides souls, brings the soul to the new clay human. On the Trinity sarcophagus, Christ, who is the shepherd of man's souls, holds something in his hand that looks like two small wings. These could refer to the butterfly wings of Psyche, or to a different mythological tradition where Athena delivers the human soul in the shape of a bird or a bee (as can be seen on a Prometheus-sarcophagus in the Capitoline Museum in Rome).

PROMETHEUS IN THE GARDEN OF EDEN

The connection between God the creator and Prometheus has been established. Towards the end of the Middle Ages, the episode of creation is the sole episode from the myth of Prometheus that can be found in art. Occasionally, the narrative is combined with story of the theft of fire, but only if the fire is then used to animate the created human. Other elements of the myth, especially the scene of Prometheus' punishment where the eagle devours his liver, appear in literary sources but were not depicted in extant images.. The connection between God the Creator and Prometheus was so evident that in some fourteenth-century manuscripts, Prometheus makes an appearance in depictions of the Christian creation story, or rather, the Christian creation myth appeared in illustrations of the myth.

The following two images are illuminations accompanying the *Ovide Moraliseé*, a retelling from ca. 1325-1350 – in old French and put to rhyme – of the *Metamorphoses* by Ovid. In a poem on the Prometheus myth, the author combines the Titan's creation of mankind out of clay with his theft of fire, which he uses to animate his creation. The poem also provides a Christian moralisation to accompany the story: humans should not try to oppose God and the will of heaven shall prevail. This Christian interpretation

Fig. 5.8 God creates the world, Prometheus animates humans, Illustration from the Ovide Moralisée, c. 1325-1350, Bibliothèque Municipale, Lyon, MS 742, fol. 4r

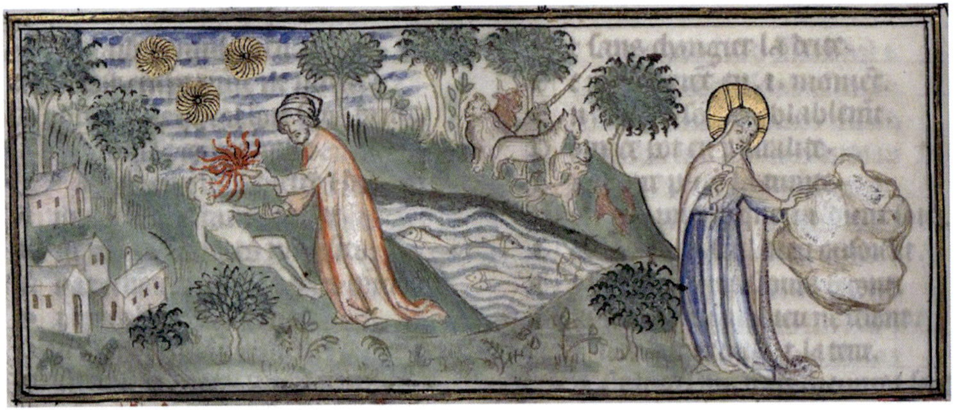

of the myth is further strengthened by the illustration that accompanies it (fig. 5.8). Here we see how the story of Prometheus is combined with the Christian tale of creation. God, depicted at the right of the image, crowned with a nimbus, creates the universe. To the left, we see Prometheus in this newly created world of plants, animals, heavenly bodies, and several houses, executed in gold leaf. The Titan uses his fennel stalk to carry the Olympic fire to earth, and bring humans to life.

A slightly later illumination in a manuscript containing the same text makes the identification of the figure as Prometheus even more explicit (fig. 5.9.). Here the biblical story of creation is depicted in four distinct phases. First, at the upper left, we see God creating earth and air out of chaos. The swirling blue and while lines at the top of the scene are a medieval narrative tool to signify the supernatural, in this case the primordial chaos that existed 'in the beginning.' On the second image, to the upper right, all animals have been created and we once again see several houses. In the bottom left, Prometheus suddenly enters the scene. Any doubt regarding his identity is taken away: his name 'Promethe' is carefully painted next to his head. With the fire of the gods, he brings Adam to life. He then passes the baton back to God, who creates Eve out of the rib of Adam.

We have seen how artists and theorists in the Middle Ages adapted classical myth to fit within Christian thought and image-making systems. This adaptation was accomplished through the appropriation of antique pictorial language to tell new Christian stories. On the other hand, they sought out thematic overlaps and similarities between Christianity and classical antiquity. Prometheus was a figure of interest for the medieval mind because of the way that he brought lifeless matter to life, which seemed to correspond with the Christian doctrine of resurrection. In addition to that the connection was made between Prometheus and God because both of them were 'creators of men'.

The joining together of body and soul recurs in medieval theories concerning the function of the liver. This shall be expanded upon in the next chapter.

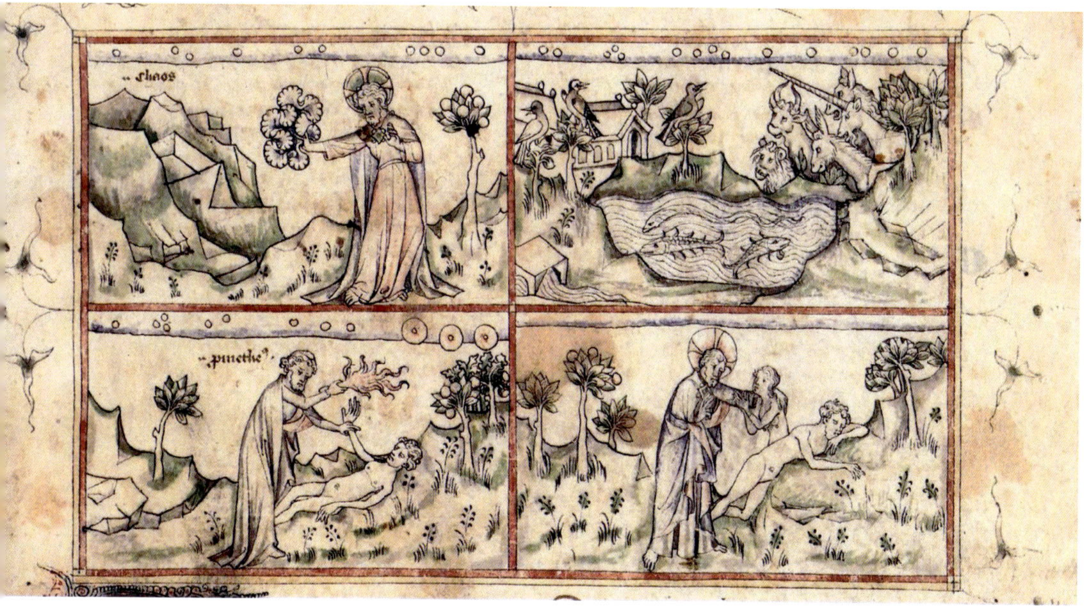

Fig. 5.9 God creates the world, Prometheus animates humans, Illustration from the Ovide Moralisée, 1375-1400, Bibliothèque Nationale, Paris, MS fr. 871, fol. 31

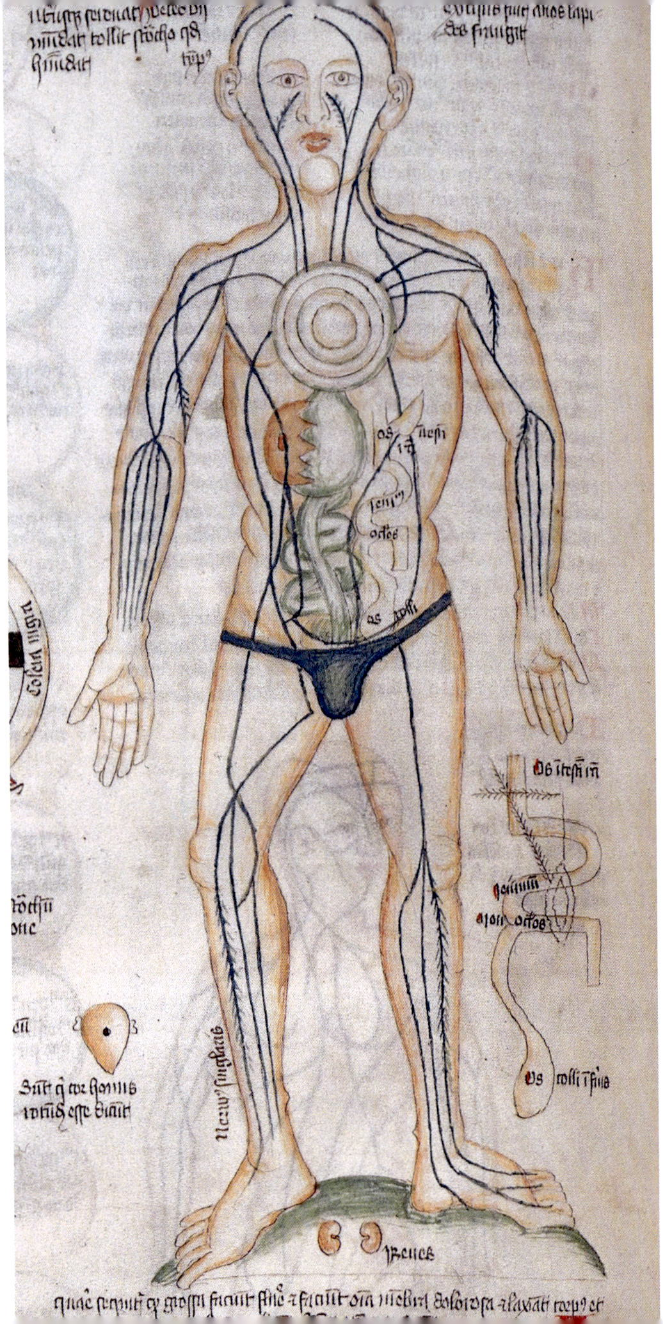
Renes

6
THE LIVER IN THE THE MIDDLE AGES, ACCORDING TO GALEN

Fig. 6.1 Portrait of Claudius Galenus (130-201 CE), Lithographic print by P.R. Vigneron, 1820-1829, Wellcome Library, London

Claudius Galen (130-201 CE), born in Pergamon, was the most respected medical authority from Graeco-Roman antiquity (fig. 6.1). His teachings, based in large part on the writings of Hippocrates and Aristotle, defined medical thought and practice for fifteen centuries. The work of Galen, as he was more commonly called, was to the field of medicine what the Bible was to the Church, and questioning it in any way was akin to heresy.

Galen studied medicine in Pergamon (modern day Bergama in north-western Turkey), after which he visited the famous medical schools in Smyrna, Corinth, and Alexandria. He finally settled in Rome where he became the personal physician of emperor Commodus and the head phy-

Fig. 6.0 'Organ man', picture from: Apocalypse, *c. 1420, 40 x 30 cm, Wellcome Library, London, MS49, fol. 36 v.*

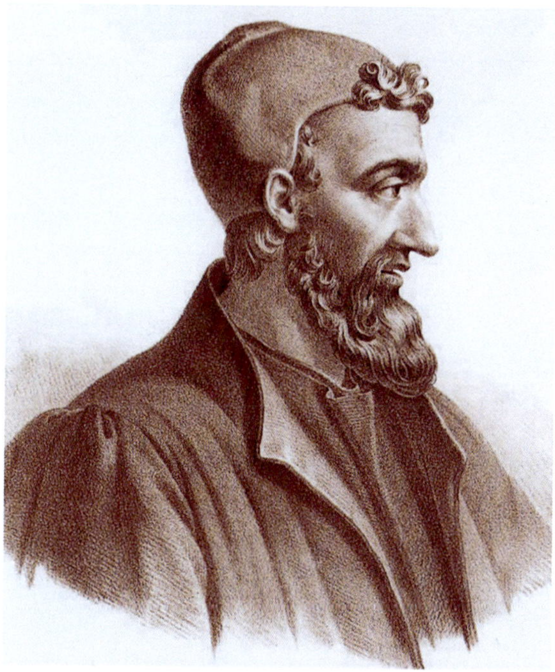

sician of the Gladiators. In Rome, he established a successful practice, as well as his own apothecary consisting of hundreds of types of plant or animal based medicine. Galen left a considerable corpus of medical works, originally written in Greek. In addition to these, he published a large number of non-medical books concerning philosophy and rhetoric. His best-known medical work is the *Ars Medica*. His foundational thought when building his medical theory is that the build and function of the human body were teleological in nature, that is to say that they were geared towards a goal or purpose, which was decided upon by the creator, the all-knowing God.

In his study of *pneuma* (air) Galen recognised three types of life force:

1) The soul-spirit (*Spiritus animalis*), that resides in the brain and nerves.
2) The life-spirit (*Spiritus vitalis*), that is created in the heart and is transported through the arteries.
3) The natural-spirit (*Spiritus naturalis*), which is produced in the liver and fills the veins. Because Galen believed that blood was produced in the liver, he equated the natural-spirit with blood from the veins.

Galen had his own ideas about the transport of blood through the body, and these remained unchallenged until the discovery of the circulatory system by William Harvey (1578-1657) in 1628. According to Galen, organs received nutrients from blood that moved back and forth through the veins, like the tides at sea. The blood was purified of pollutants in the lungs, which were exhaled. It subsequently found it's way from the right to the left chamber of the heart through 'pores' in the cardiac septum. This is also where the 'pneuma' ended up that was extracted from the air by the lungs. In the left chamber of the heart, the pneuma reacted with the 'inner warmth' (*calor innatus*) and made the blood bubble and foam, after which the heart expanded and the foaming blood would follow its journey through the arteries. This dogma on the movement of blood persisted for centuries and was treated as the sole certainty by European anatomists. This blind belief was so strong that anatomists, when doing dissections of the heart, perforated the cardiac septum dividing the right and left chambers of the heart themselves in order to uphold Galen's theories.

Galen saw the heart as the origin of the arteries, and the liver as the centre for the veins. The *Porta hepatis* on the lowerside of the liver was the place where the veins of the intestines were gathered through the portal vein. Blood would be formed in the liver – a reasonable conclusion given how saturated with blood the organ is. The liver had three important functions within Galen's theory: it secreted bile; it radiated heat; and it stored nutrients. Galen had, however, never seen a proper representation of a human liver, due to the? fact that the practice of dissecting bodies was very limited during his lifetime. While he did produce detailed reports of dissections, these had been conducted on animals (mainly pigs), whose liver he studied and recorded. In pigs, the liver has five lobes, and because of this, some representations of the liver in the Middle Ages show the organ with five lobes.

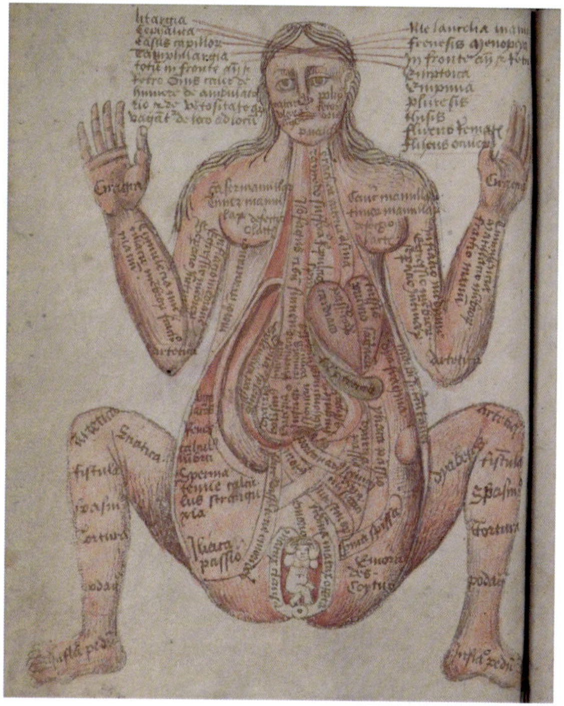

Fig. 6.2 Pseudo-Galenus, Anatomia, *England, mid-15th-century, Wellcome Library, London*

Galen's teachings were the leading texts until well into the Middle Ages and his works were translated into Latin and Arabic—the latter by the Persian doctor Avicenna (980-1037). His *Canon Medicinae*, or 'Canon of medicine,' was the standard medical text in the Middle East for centuries, gaining him the epithet 'the Arabic Galen.' It is remarkable that Galen's works, and all medical treatises following them, did not contain many anatomical illustrations. This shows how limited a physician's practical knowledge of the human body really was. In later reproductions of his books, this particular one dating from the mid-15th century, one can find a depiction of a pregnant woman (fig. 6.2). The liver is depicted central in the illustration with its lobes and a green gallbladder.

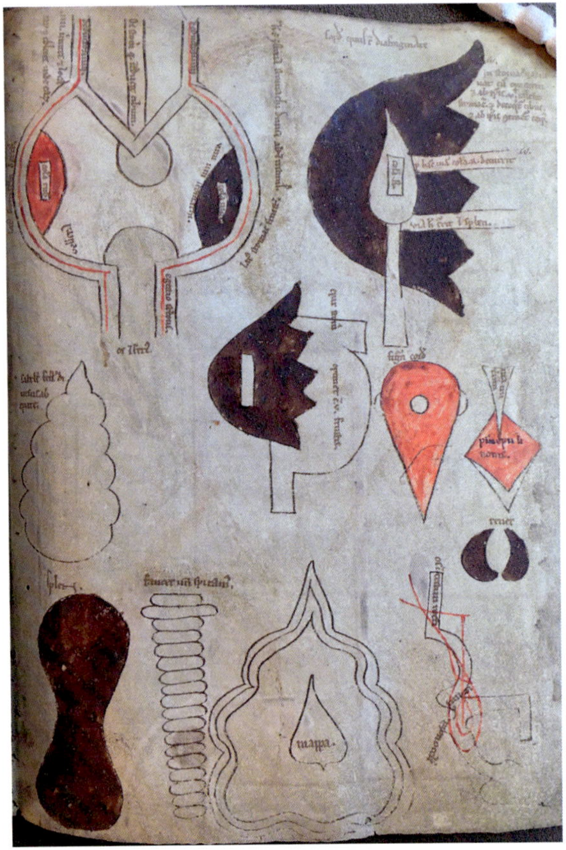

The oldest medieval depiction of the liver can be found in an English manuscript from the twelfth century, now kept in the library at Gonville and Caius College, Cambridge (fig. 6.3). In this manuscript, we find the earliest known depictions of the organs in the abdominal cavity, schematically portrayed in stylised linework. In the upper left corner of the compoisition, we see the stomach divided in four compartments to represent the four humours; red and black bile are coloured in and placed on either side of the stomach. Underneath the illustration of the stomach, we see the liver, with five lobes, depicted in dark brown. The contour that surrounds it is the stomach and the rectangular shape that is left blank in the centre signifies the position of the gallbladder. In the upper right corner, we see another, more detailed depiction of the liver and gallbladder, its pear-shape more faithfully depicted. There are three channels leading to the organ responsible for the transport of red bile. The red, teardrop-shaped organ beneath the liver is meant to represent the heart, flanked by two 'auricles', ear like structures extending from the hart. Comparable depictions of the stomach, liver and gallbladder can be found in the *Apocalypse*, an illustrated text that appeared ca. 1420 (fig. 6.0).

In the high Middle Ages, Mondino de' Luzzi (1275-1326), an Italian anatomist-surgeon from Bologna, produced a book meant for the study of anatomy that for two centuries dictated anatomical knowledge (*Anatomia Mundini*, 1316). De' Luzzi's anatomical

Fig. 6.3 Illustration of separately depicted organs in the abdominal cavity, 12th-century English manuscript, Codex Caius 223/190. Gonville and Caius College, Cambridge

descriptions were based on observations made during the dissection of human corpses. As can be seen in Figure 6.4, the liver (D) was conventionally depicted with five lobes. De' Luzzi identified two large veins that originate from the liver: the portal vein (*vena porta*) on the underside of the liver and the *vena cava* from the top of the right lobe. The bile duct with the gallbladder (E) is depicted as connecting to the *duodenum* (F), where he describes the finding of an extra bile duct that leads to the stomach (B). It is possible that De' Luzzi misidentified the left liver artery (*Arteria hepatica sinistra*) that sometimes springs forth from the left stomach artery (*Arteria gastrica sinistra*) as an extra bile duct (fig. 6.4).

Hence, not much was known of the liver in the dark Middle Ages as most organs were veiled in darkness too. Because of the lack of dissections, anatomical insights were missing and knowledge of liver morphology only fragmentary.

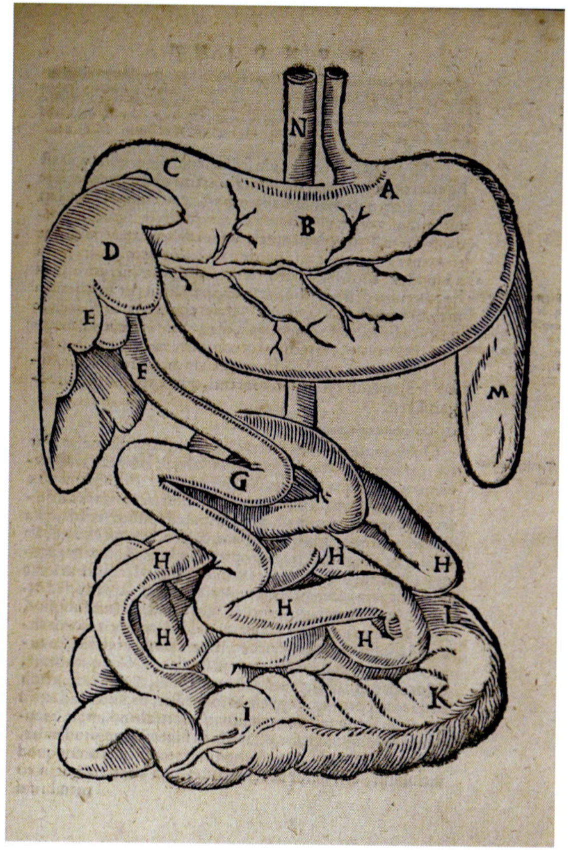

Fig. 6.4 Illustration of organs of the abdominal cavity, Anatomia Mundini, *Mondino de' Luzzi (1275-1326), 1475, Padua*

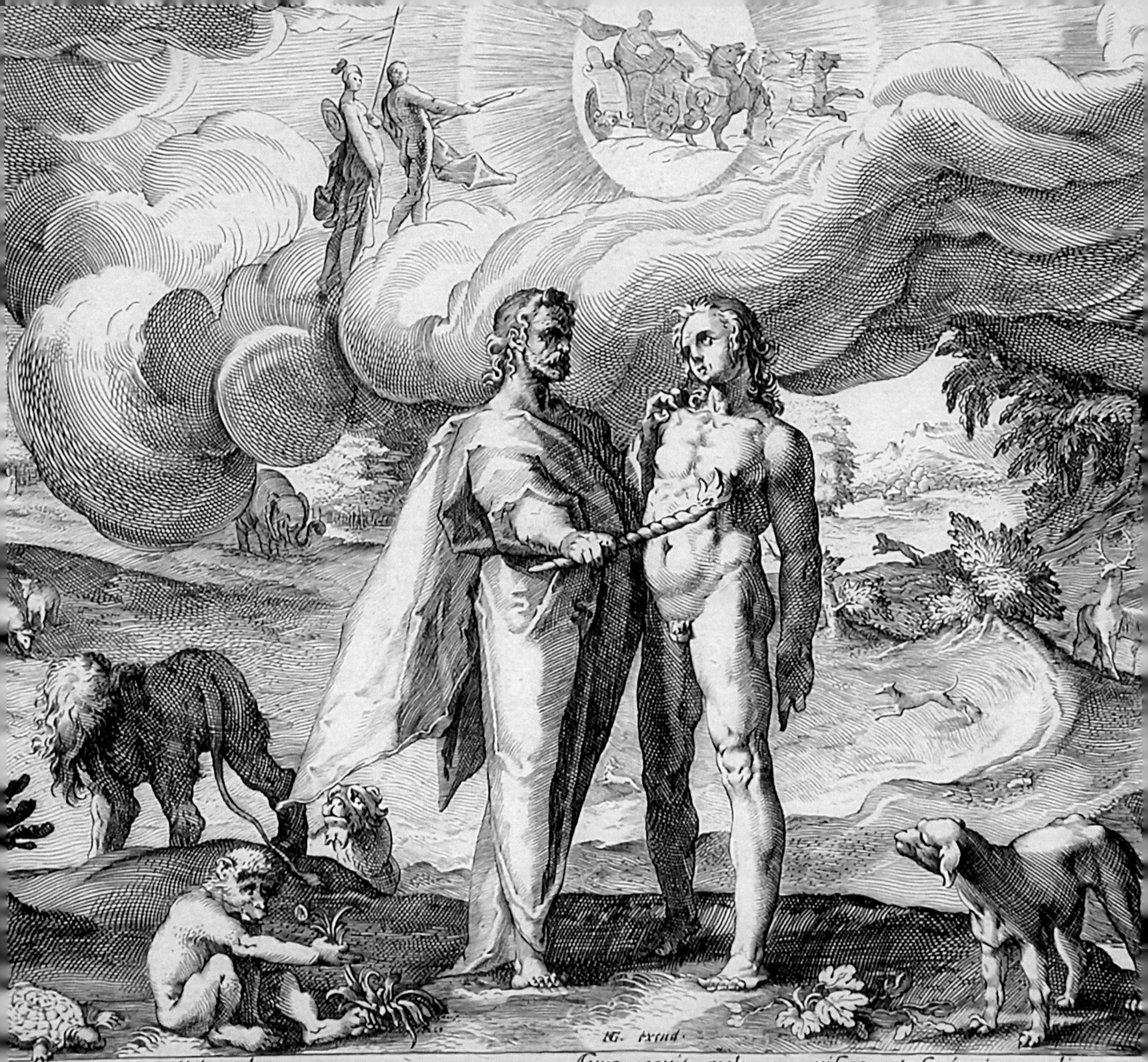

…certos secreuit in orbes … Aura, capit volucres, pisces versantur in vndis,

7

PROMETHEUS IN THE RENAISSANCE

Fig. 7.0 Hendrick Goltzius, Prometheus creates the first human and steals the heavenly fire in a paradisical garden filled with animals. Engraving, c. 1589, 176 × 252mm, Rijksmuseum, Amsterdam

Renaissance means 'rebirth.' In the period of ca. 1453 to 1600, an interplay of political, economic and cultural circumstances facilitated a tremendous flourishing of the arts and sciences. People found a renewed interest in classical antiquity, and this is strongly reflected in the art from this period. The term 'rebirth' refers to this rekindled interest. In these one hundred and fifty years, the figure and myth of Prometheus also underwent a rebirth in kind.

Through the course of the late Middle Ages, new texts from classical antiquity were reintroduced in Western Europe. These texts had been preserved in Islamic countries, while they were lost to the Christian West. The reintroduction of these texts produced a considerable new corpus of source materials that western scholars could concern themselves with. Certain impactful events contributed to the reintroduction of these texts: despite their military character, the crusades had increased exposure to and contact with Islamic countries in the Levant, creating trading routes between West and East, Christian and Muslim. During the same period, the campaigns of the Reconquista, the conquest of Spain my Christian powers, were gradually opening up contact with Islamic Spain, which started the slow influx of new texts. One event was most impactful of all: The fall of Constantinople in 1453. Not only did the fall cause an influx of Byzantine Greek refugees—among whom

Fig. 7.1 Page from a Florentine picture chronicle featuring both biblical figures and figures from classical mythology. Here we see Inachus, Prometheus and 'king Pharaoh'. Prometheus is dressed in the robes of a scholar or astronomer, while holding a small figure of a human in his raised hand. With a stylus he provides the finishing touches for his work. School of Maso Finiguerra, 1470-1475, brown ink and charcoal on paper, 32,7 x 23,8 mm, British Museum, London

were many scholars, eagerly employed by Italian elites— but the event also precipitated the establishment of an intensive and profitable trade relationship between Italy and the Ottoman empire. The influx of these tets meant an increased exposure to previously unknown ancient mythology and philosophy. However, in the Christian West the study of 'pagan' mythology and philosophy still had to be justified.

In the chapter 5, we saw that, after the fall of the Roman Empire, Prometheus – a Pagan deity – became embedded in the realm of Christian thought. The Christian appropriation of the myth was justified because parallels could be made between Prometheus and God as creators of mankind. Prometheus' story became a *genesis secundum gentiles* (a genesis according to the pagans). Another practice that justified Christian writing on myths was to provide them with a rationalistic reading—a practice that was already established within the ancient world, where scholars sometimes found such fantastic tales incompatible with their own common sense. In these so-called 'Euhemeristic' readings, a historical source was sought to explain the origin of the myth. One example of such a reading would be the explanation for the mythical centaur—a creature that, in a euhemerist interpretation, was thought to be based on Scythian warriors who had first perfected warfare on horseback. Another way to establish a type of reality for myths was to interpret them as allegorical stories. Both of these methods for rationalising mythology were eagerly adopted by the Christian West, in order to make sense of the stories. Rationalising these stories enabled scholars to treat them as valuable sources without the risk of presenting them as religious texts.

EUHEMERISM AND THE SEARCH FOR A HISTORICAL PROMETHEUS

The myth of Prometheus was not exempt from euhemerist interpretation. Several authors proposed possible historical origins for the myth. Servius (born 363 CE) identified Prometheus as an Assyrian astrologer who, from the high precipice of the Caucasian mountains, studied the stars, after which he descended to share his astrological knowledge with mankind. His torment, according to Servius, was the torment of possessing a

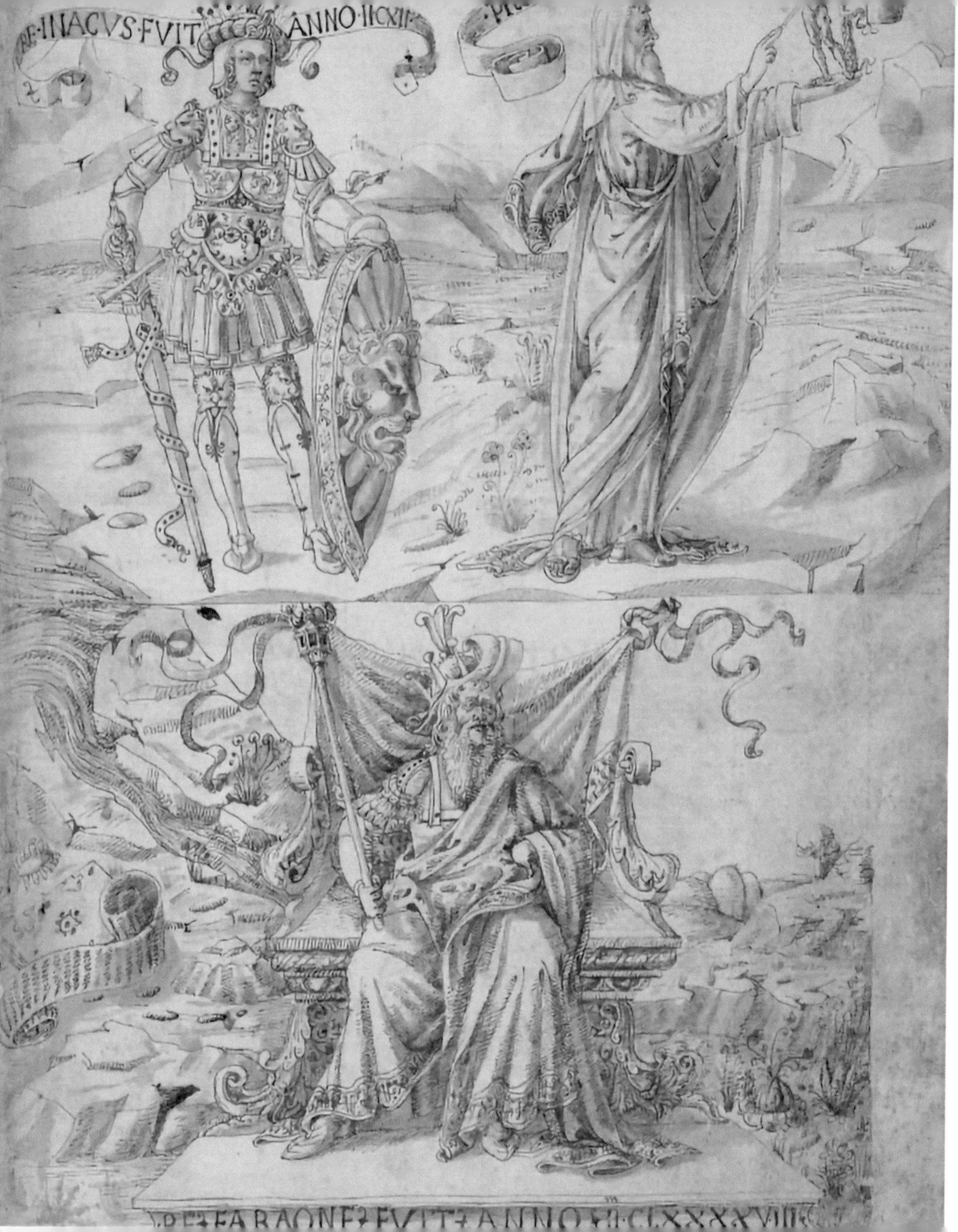
RE·INACVS·FVIT ANNO·IICXII
RE FARAONE FVIT ANNO CLXXXXVIII

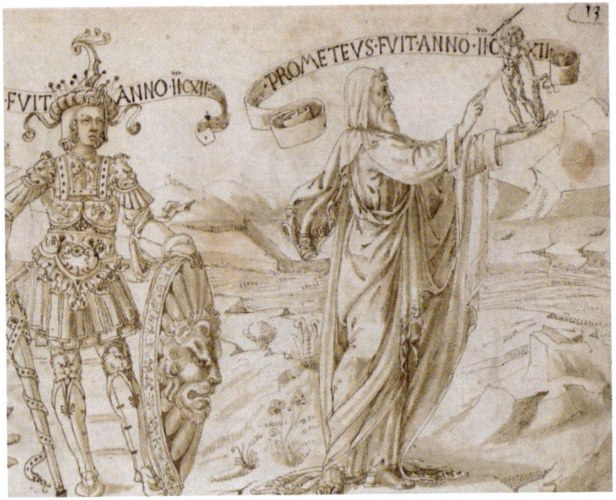

Fig. 7.2 Page from a Florentine picture chronicle (Detail of Fig. 7.1)

great mind that plagues all big thinkers. The stealing of the Olympic fire could then be explained as Prometheus discovering the origin of lightning.

In this manner, Prometheus became a historical figure—an actual person who many believed to have truly lived. He was historically situated in the 'third age of the world' (that according to the *aetates mundi* – the six Biblical ages of the world – lasted from the life and rule of Abraham to that of David). Due to a linguistic mishap, some texts suggest that Prometheus was the son of Japheth, one of the sons of Noah. This designation was the result of the similarity between the names Japheth and Iapetus, Prometheus' mythic father and the son of the primal gods Uranus and Gaia. Prometheus was also connected to the biblical story about the first sculptor, who lived in the third age. This sculptor was so talented, and his sculptures so lifelike, that his work gave rise to the birth of idolatry and so-called less intelligent humans revered him as a god. Some interpretations suggest that Prometheus was this biblical sculptor. Because of this historization, Prometheus is increasingly found in genealogical texts. These texts contained descriptions of family trees and dynasties, often featuring biblical, mythological and historical figures. Italy produced an illustrated tradition of such books called the picture chronicles.

One such picture chronicle can be found in the British Museum in London (fig. 7.1). It was published in ca. 1470-1475 in Florence and consists of fifty-three full plates that show both biblical and mythological figures in chronological order. The delicate pen and ink drawings are probably from the school of Maso Finiguerra (1426-1464). The book does not contain any text, save lines from text scrolls on which the names and dates associated with the figures depicted are listed.

The image shows, from left to right and from top to bottom, King Inachus, Prometheus and 'King Pharaoh.' The last was the pharaoh from the story of Moses; however, the context and meaning of the term 'pharaoh' was unknown to medieval and renaissance audiences and was thus read as a proper name. Prometheus is dressed as an ancient philosopher and holds a small statue in his hand that he is in the act of sculpting with a *stilus*. These figures originate in a wide range of sources, but are depicted together because they were believed to all hail from the same biblical time period (the third age).

PROMETHEUS THE HOMO DOCTUS, AN ALLEGORY FOR SCHOLARS

In the previous section, we saw that the Prometheus story was given a euhemerist reading, but he was also provided with an allegorical interpretation. This was given to him by the famous Italian poet Boccaccio (1313-1375) *Della genealogiaa deorum gentilium*, which he composed in 1360. This book was dedicated to unfurling the complex familiar relations of the Greco-Roman pantheon. Boccaccio begins by recounting the famous Prometheus myth, but adds an episode to the story of Epimetheus, Prometheus' brother and the Titan god of hindsight, which the author drew from various sources that he had combined. He wrote that Epimetheus crafted a statue as well, but that this displeased Zeus to such an extent that he destroyed the statue and turned Epimetheus into a monkey in punishment. Boccacccio also makes important changes where Prometheus is concerned. In his edition of the text, it is not Prometheus' liver that is torn out by the eagle, but his heart. Boccaccio's Titan also steals the fire from the flaming chariot of Apollo, rather than from Hephaistus' forge.

The Renaissance began earlier in Italy than it did in the rest of Europe, and Bocaccio's allegorical reading of Prometheus indeed shows an early spark of Renaissance thought. The allegorical explanation of the Prometheus myth exists in two parts. The first is very straightforward; Boccaccio reads Prometheus as a symbol of the true God, who also created a human out of clay. The second explanation utilises the above-mentioned rationalist explanation in which Prometheus is an Assyrian astrologist. Boccaccio explains that the story of Prometheus must be read as an exemplary tale that scholars could mirror. The story has three different iterations of man; initially, we find humans in their natural state, the *homo naturalis*. Prometheus is the *homo doctus*, the enlightened human, and it is through his help that mankind is elevated out of this *homo naturalis* stage and able to form a civilised life as the *homo civilis*. This concept of the *homo doctus* was an important new ideal that rose to prominence in the Renaissance and served as the highest standard for scholars. Thus, scholars began to identify with Prometheus, an alignment that is reflected in images from this period. This is in strong contrast with the Middle Ages where the myth was only included insofar as the superiority of the Christian faith could be showcased. It is through the influence of Boccaccio that Prometheus regained philosophical appreciation as the embodiment of the ideal of *homo doctus*.

This self-identification of scholars with Prometheus is reflected in the *Neurenberg chronicle*, a woodcarving produced in Germany and published by Hartmann Schedel (1440-1514) in 1493 (fig. 7.3). Here, Prometheus is included as a descendant of Zeus. We see him wearing the German robes of a *Magister Scholae* (a very learned man) after which the robes of current academics are still modelled. He is holding a ring, in reference to Aeschylus' text in which the invention of rings is included in the long list of skills taught to mankind by Prometheus. It was a popular euhemerist explanation to identify Prometheus as the inventor of rings, where the myth was a fantasy surrounding an everyday inventor.

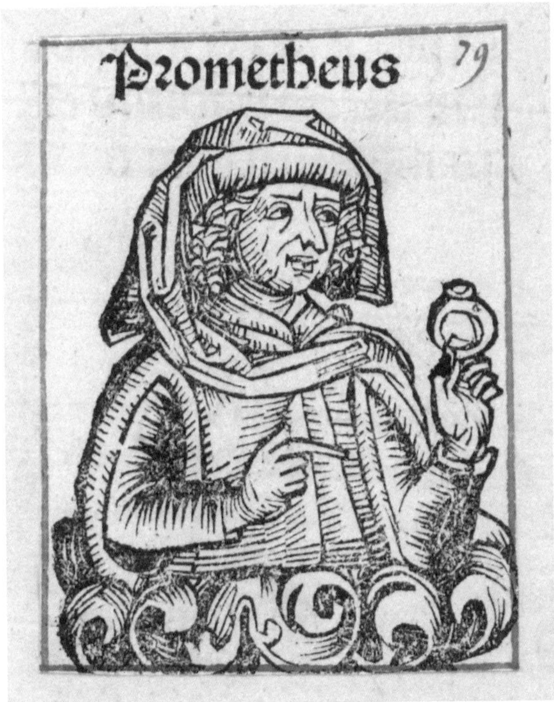

Fig. 7.3 Prometheus dressed as a 'Magister Scholae', Woodcarving in the Nurenberg chronicles by Hartmann Schedel (school of Michel Wogemut), 1493, h. 62 × w. 48 mm, Rijksmuseum Amsterdam

The Renaissance found a new love for a type of painting: the allegory. In an allegorical picture, multiple figures from classical mythology are depicted together to convey a message that a learned audience could decipher. Prometheus as archetype of reason and science finds its apex in the *Studiolo*, the study, of Francesco I de' Medici (1541-1587). Medici commissioned the *Studiolo* to be constructed at the Palazzo Vecchio in Florence. Small cupboards were installed all along the walls of the Studiolo, and functioned as cabinets of curiosities containing scientific instruments. All available surfaces were covered in paintings that played together as one large allegory. It was a true *Wunderkammer*. The famous painter, architect, and theorist Giorgio Vasari (1511-1574) designed the complex decorative program and it was completed between 1570 and 1575. The scholars Vicenzo Borghini and Batista Adriani, along with Vasari, supervised the team of well-known artists hired to bring to life in paint the variety of myths depicted. On the four walls, we see fourty-four different scenes related to the four elements: fire, water, earth and air. Each element is represented through depictions of different crafts and inventions associated with individual elements. Examples include the casting of bronze for fire, blowing glass for air, excavating gold for earth, and fishing for pears for water. This entire allegory cumulates in the central fresco on the ceiling (fig. 7.4). Here, the personification of nature offers gold and fire to Prometheus, the father of all arts. Prometheus is not categorised in the section of the element of fire, like one might expect. The fire of Prometheus is not an earthly or 'elemental' fire; he instead possesses a 'spiritual' fire that surpasses above the elements.

PROMETHEUS AS A PUZZLE: DECIPHERING AN ALLEGORY

The emphasis on Prometheus as an example for scholars has also led to instances where his story was depicted independently of other canonical myths.

One example of a Prometheus allegory can be found on two *cassoni* painted by Piero di Cosimo (1462-1522). A *cassone* is an Italian bridal chest that was often given by the bride's family to the bride as marriage present. The large frontal panels of the chests were often painted, as is the case for these two *cassoni*. On these *cassoni,* Piero di Cosimo has painted multiple scenes from the Prometheus myth in the same picture plane, in a practice called 'continuous narrative.' The complexity of the allegory becomes clear when we take a closer look at the works and attempt to identify all the figures.

On the first cassone, created in 1515 and now in the Alte Pinakothek in Munich (fig. 7.5), we see four scenes from the myth. Easiest to identify is the scene in the upper-right corner, where we see Prometheus being carried to heaven by Athena to steal the fire from

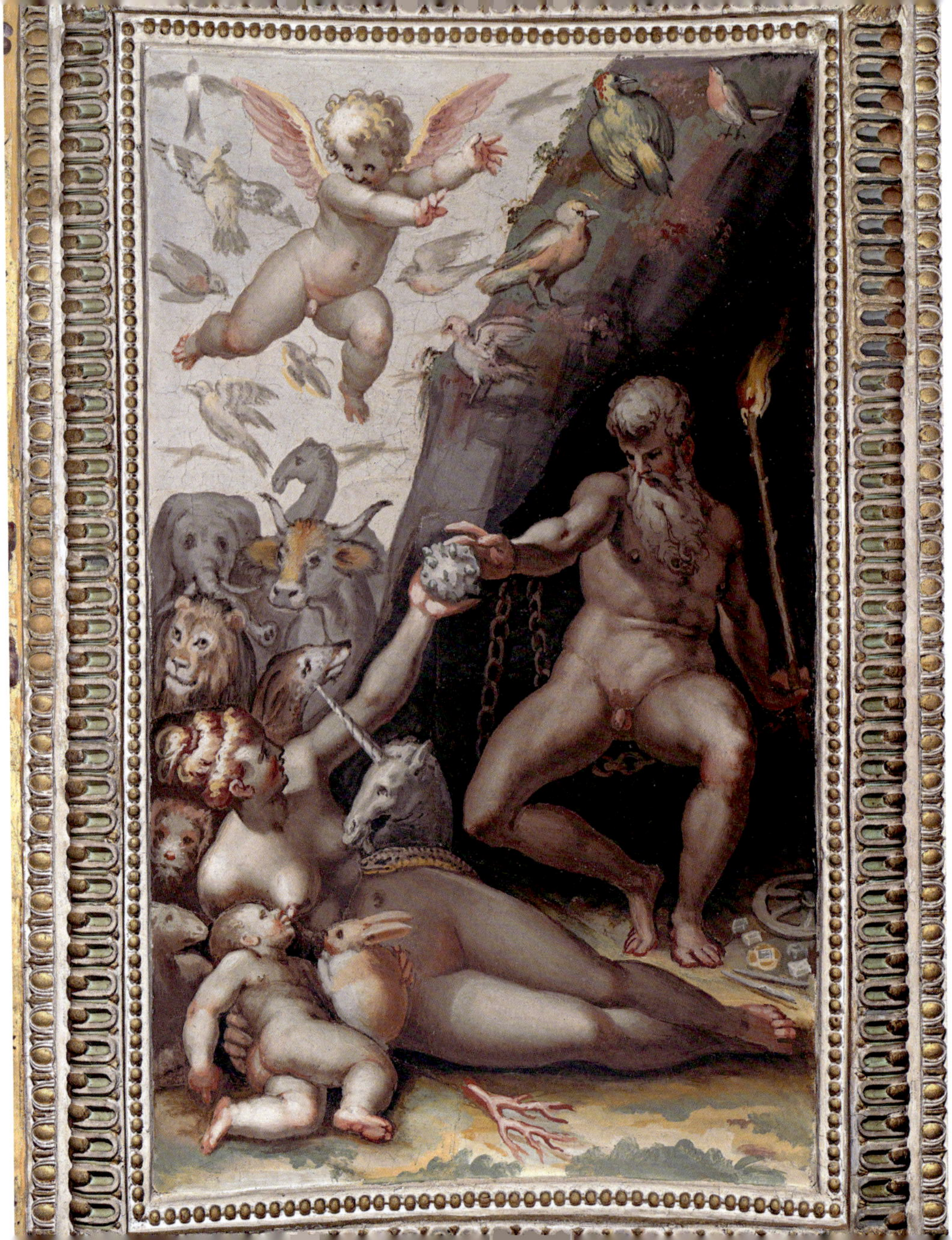

Fig. 7.4 Nature offers fire and gold to Prometheus, father of all arts, central ceiling painting in the studiolo of Francesco I de' Medici, 1572, Fresco, Palazzo Vecchio, Florence

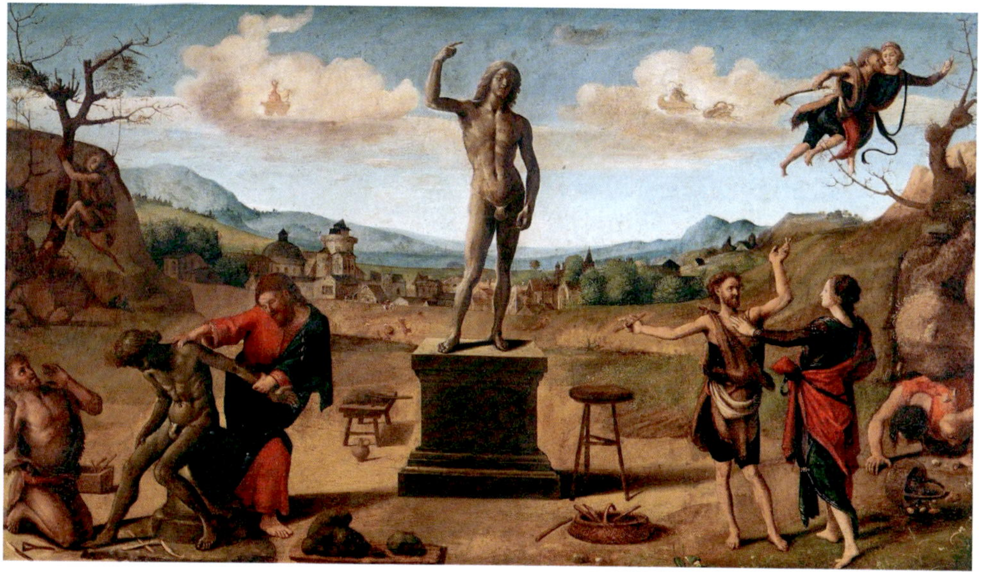

Fig. 7.5 Piero di Cosimo, cassone with a Prometheus allegory. Bottom left: Zeus destroys the statue made by Epimetheus. Upper left: Epimetheus is punished and turned into a monkey. Bottom right: Athena praises Prometheus' craftsmanship. Upper right: Athena and Prometheus ascend heavenward with a fennel stalk. 1515, oil paint on wood, 66 x 118,7 cm. Alte Pinakothek, Munich

the chariot of the sun. Prometheus is dressed in a black tunic with a brown toga and the white apron of an artisan, and he is consistently shown wearing these clothes throughout all the scenes. He is clearly identifiable through the fennel stalk that he holds in his hand.

We once again see the figures of Athena and Prometheus together at the bottom-right of the composition. Prometheus is proudly gesturing to the statue of a man with the *stilus* still in his hand, the statue stands proudly in the center of the painting. Athena praises his craftsmanship by putting her hand on his shoulder.

The scene on the bottom-left is harder to interpret. We see a second statue of a human made from clay. The clay gleams, as though it is still wet, and lumps of raw clay are piled on the floor next to the statue. It is clearly a different statue from the one made by Prometheus – the central statue has long hair that reaches past the shoulders, while the seated statue has

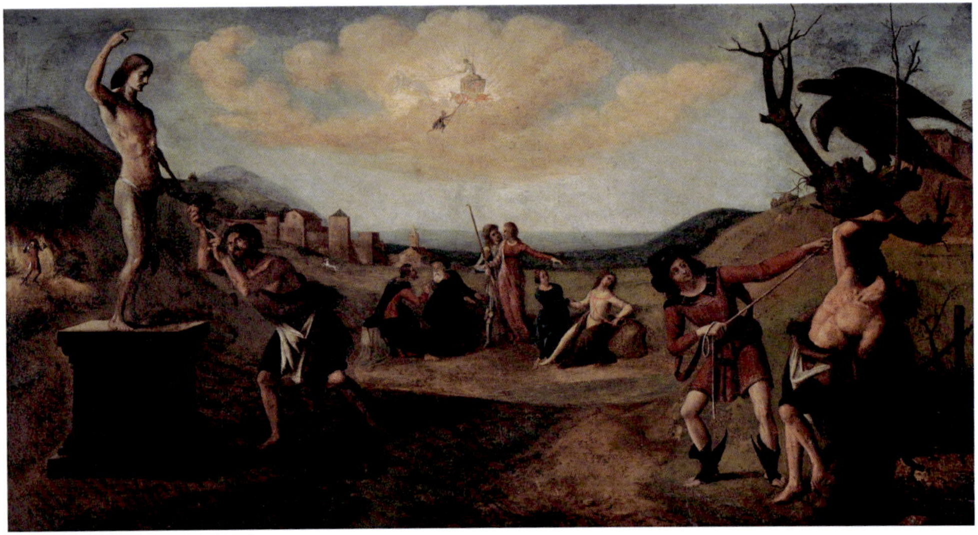

Fig. 7.6 Piero di Cosimo, cassone with a Prometheus allegory. Upper middle: Prometheus steals the fire from the chariot of the sun and uses it to animate his statue (bottom left). Centre: The council of the gods convenes and creates Pandora. Bottom right: Hermes ties Prometheus to a tree to receive his punishment. 1515, Oil paint on wood, 64 x 116 cm. Musée des Beaux-Arts, Strasbourg

short locks. It is possible that Piero di Cosimo was closely following Boccaccio's narration of the myth, in which Epimetheus first made a statue of man, an act that angered Zeus to such an extent that he changed Epimetheus into a monkey. This would suggest that the man who is sitting kneeled on the floor with his arms raised in indignation is Epimetheus. The brown tunic of a coarse material that hangs of his shoulders is found again in a figure that is climbing a tree in the upper-left part of the scene – a figure with the tail and facial features of a monkey. Indeed, it is the transformed Epimetheus who glances over his shoulder, looking back at the previous scene at the bottom-left of the composition.

Who, then, is the figure in red and blue with long hair that is manhandling the clay sculpture and what is he doing with it? The appearance of this figure—the beard, the shoulder-length hair, the colours and style of the mantle—show strong similarities with contemporary depictions of Christ and God the Father. It is unlikely that we are looking at the Christian God here; this is most likely the mythic god Zeus taking on the characteristics associated with a 'supreme deity.' This may therefore be the scene where Zeus destroys the sculpture made by Epimetheus, which would explain the shocked expression on Epimetheus' face. A different interpretation of the same scene is that we *are* looking at the Christian God, and that this was Piero di Cosimo's attempt at depicting the first allegorical explanation of Boccaccio's retelling of the Prometheus myth. This retelling describes God as the 'first Prometheus,' the one to create the first human, the *homo naturalis*, who Prometheus subsequently elevated to become the *homo civilis*. The human clay sculpture in the natural state bends down towards the earth, while the civilised man made by Prometheus points up towards the heavens. The complexity of the image and the different possible readings was intentioned, inviting a learned public to try and solve the image as though it were a puzzle and have discussions on its deeper meaning.

The story is continued in the second *cassone*, also produced in 1515 and now in the Musée des Beaux-Arts in Strasbourg (fig. 7.6). The scenes on this panel prove to be even harder to interpret. The narrative begins in the centre-top of the painting. While he ascended to the heavens in the previous painting, it is only here that we see Prometheus stealing the fire. The chariot is shining with bright rays of light, and in the clouds, Prometheus holds his fennel stalk in the flaming chariot wheels. In the left-front of the panel Prometheus presses the torch with the stolen fire against the chest of his statue—the same statue as depicted in the first *cassone*—and thus bringing it to life. To the right, we see the consequences that befell Prometheus for this theft Hermes, clad in Renaissance clothing but still recognisable by his winged boots, ties the Titan to a tree, where the eagle is hungrily awaiting him.

The difficulty in interpretation arises when we turn our attention to the group of figures in the centre of the painting (fig. 7.7). These figures may be the council of the gods creating Pandora. This explanation is enforced by the reappearance of the Christ-like Zeus in red and blue at the far left, who instructs the other gods in Pandora's creation. The old man and the women in red would then be Saturn and Aphrodite. These fig-

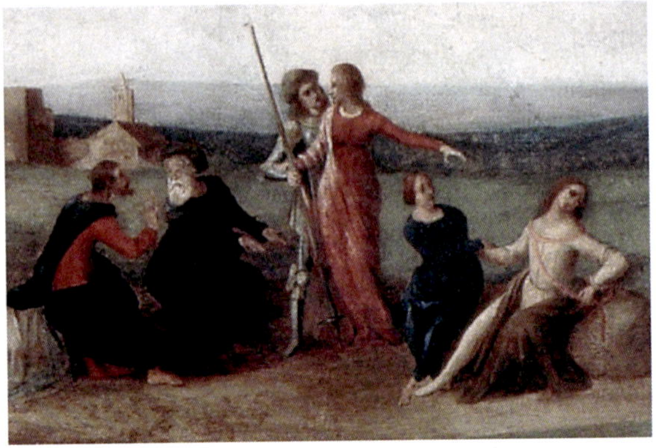

Afb. 7.7 Piero di Cosimo, The council of the gods convenes and creates Pandora (detail of fig. 7.6)

ures are identifiable when compared with the other *cassone* panel illustrations, which show two chariots in the sky, one pulled by winged serpents and the other by doves—attributes of the two gods, respectively. The man in armour may be Hermes, in his guise as 'slayer of Argos,' as in his epithet in Hesiodos. We propose, however, that this is Ares, the god of war, who is traditionally depicted in armour. This argument is strengthened by the way he lovingly embraces Aphrodite, given that these two gods were lovers. Finally, all figures have consistently been depicted as wearing the same clothing between different scenes and even between the two panels. Hermes has been reliably depicted in red and black clothing (as we see in the scene where he ties Prometheus to the tree, as well as the small figure in the background to the far left, behind the animated statue). This small background scene shows a different myth concerning Hermes. He is shown using a staff to separate two fighting snakes, which is how he obtained his attribute, the *caduceus*, or herald's staff: a staff encircled by two snakes. We see Athena again, extending her hand to a woman clad in white, to the far right, who would be Pandora. Aphrodite uses her extended hand to pour grace over her, while Athena offers her a shining girdle to ornate her.

It is probable that Piero di Cosimo wanted to use this *cassone* to portray the two punishments of Prometheus as the consequences of his hubris. These punishments are the torture by the eagle and the coming of Pandora. In this *cassone* painting, Pandora isn't sent to Epimetheus, but to humanity. We see that Piero di Cosimo doesn't only reference the widespread retellings and interpretations of the myth but also adopts a scene directly from Hesiodos, a classical source.

THE CLASSICS REDISCOVERED

During the course of the Renaissance, we increasingly see instances where artists or their patrons make the decision, when creating a decorative plan for an image or image cycle, to directly draw on classical sources. One example of this for the Prometheus myth can be found in a fresco by Maso Garofalo, painted on a ceiling in the Seminario Arcivescovile in Ferrara, Italy (fig. 7.8). A detail on the complex ceiling shows us Prometheus. Here, he is chained to rocks along a seashore, where he is visited by Oceanus. The traditional wall of rock is placed at the seaside in this fresco. This was probably done so that the sea god could rise up from the waves – his domain – to visit Prometheus. This scene doesn't know a visual prototype but seems to instead draw directly from the play by Aeschylus as mentioned in Chapter 3. In Aeschylus' story, Prometheus is visited by the Nereids, the daughters of the sea god Oceanus, who take pity on the Titan and then beg their father to mediate between Zeus and Prometheus. Oceanus visits Prometheusand urges him to apologise to Zeus and beg

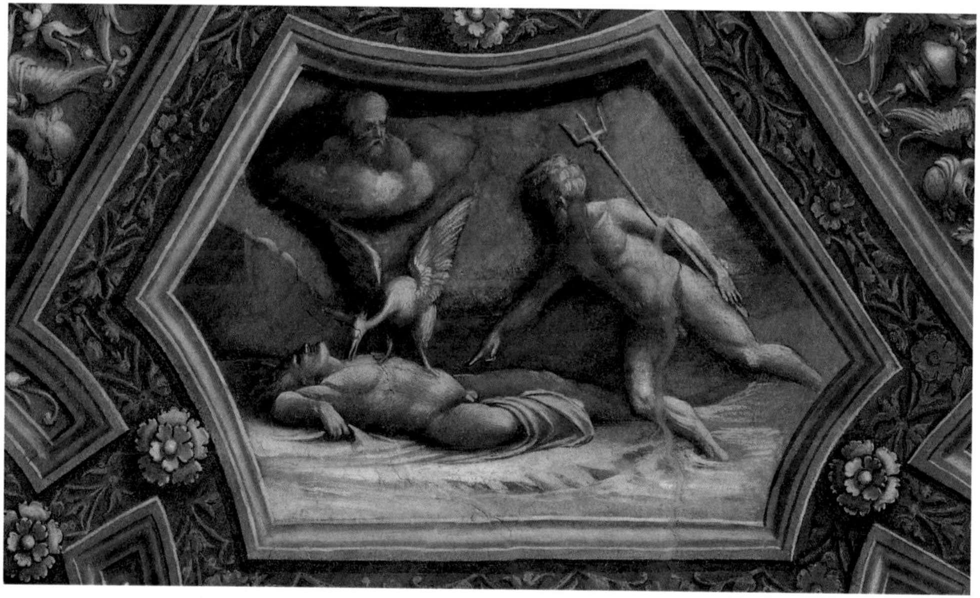

Afb. 7.8 Maso Garofalo, Detail of a fresco adorning the ceiling. Prometheus is chained on the shoreline while the eagle attacks his chest. He is visited by the sea god Oceanos. 1540, Fresco, Seminario Arcivescoville, Ferrara

Afb. 7.9 Alessandro Alciato, Woodcut of Promethues found in a book of emblems, produced in Leiden by Officina Plantiniana. Prometheus lies chained to a rock. On his stomach stands the eagle who has torn open his body. 1591, woodcut, University Library, Glasgow

for his forgiveness, foregoing his pride. Prometheus, however, refuses in a dignified manner and discloses that he knows a secret about the future that will bring about the downfall of Zeus and end his suffering. He sends Oceanus away to spare him from the damage to his reputation that suspicion of fraternising with the fallen Titan would bring him.

A CAUTIONARY TALE OF HUBRIS, PROMETHEUS CRITICISED

Outside of these scholarly environments, in which patrons idolised Prometheus, the Renaissance also knew a much more critical interpretation of the figure. In so-called Emblem books, especially popular outside of Italy, Prometheus was a symbol for hubris and pride. These types of books contained woodcuts or engravings that were accompanied by a short text in rhyme with a moralising message. The emblem book of Alessandro Alciato from 1531 is one of the books in which Prometheus figures as a cautionary tale (fig. 7.9). Prometheus has been demoted from a noble philosopher to an arrogant astrologist. The rhyme that accompanies him reads:

CAUCASIA aeternùm pendens in rupe Prometheus
Diripitur sacri praepetis ungue iecur.
Et nollet fecisse hominem: figulósque perosus
Accensam rapto damnat ab igne facem.
Roduntur variis prudentum pectora curis,
Qui caeli affectant scire, deûmque vices.

Prometheus, forever dangling from the Caucasian rock,
Is torn by the liver by the claws of the holy bird.
And wishes he'd never made humans, and while he hates those who clay
He curses the torch, lit with stolen fire
The hearts of those who look ahead are plagued by worries,
The seers that strive to know the heavens and the whims of the gods.

Quæ supra nos, nihil ad nos.

EMBLEMA CII.

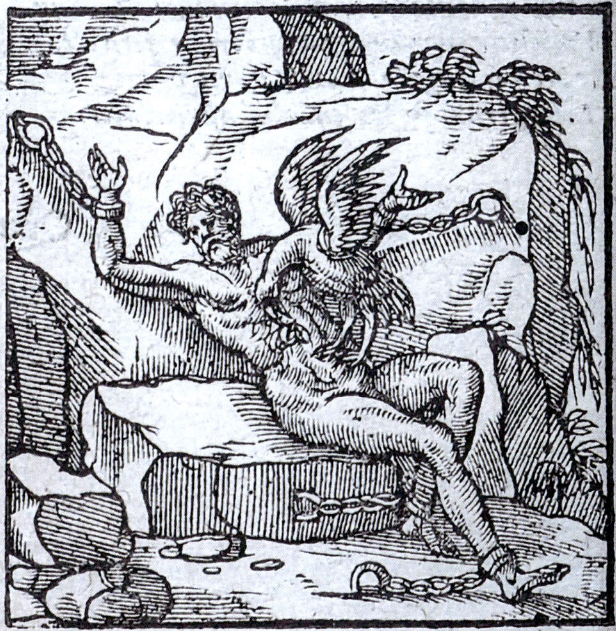

Cavcasia æternùm pẽdens in rupe Prometheus
Diripitur sacri præpetis ungue iecur.
Et nollet fecisse hominem: figulósque perosus
Accensam rapto damnat ab igne facem.
Roduntur variis prudentum pectora curis,
Qui cæli affectant scire, deûmque vices.

In astro

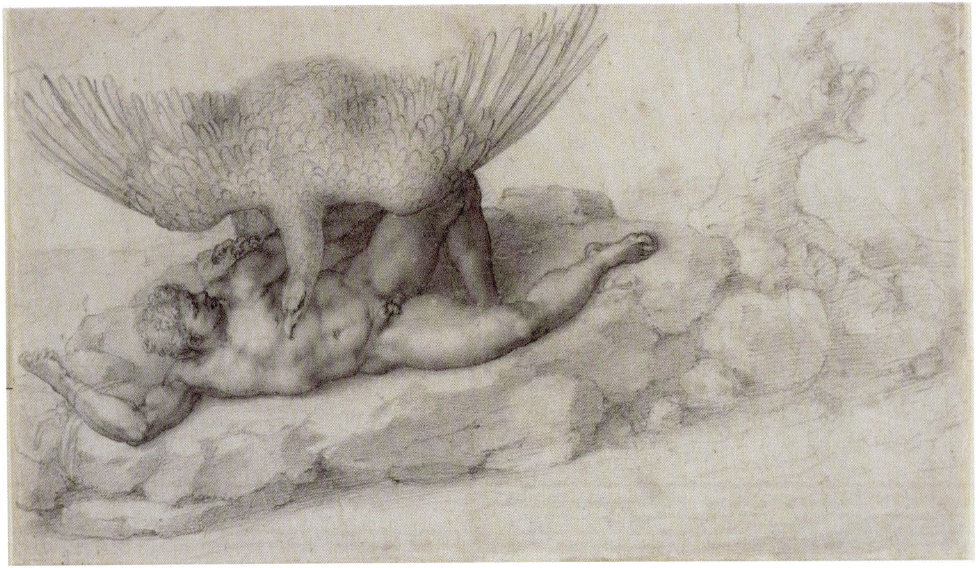

Fig. 7.10 Michelangelo Buonarotti, The punishment of Tityus. Tityus lies chained in the underworld while an eagle descends upon him to eat his liver, 1533, Drawing in black chalk, 212 x 327 mm. The Royal Library, London

The message is clear: curiosity killed the cat.

TITYUS AND THE TORTURED IMAGE

A new type of image is introduced in the Prometheus iconography, through a drawing by Michelangelo (1475-1564) from 1533 now in the Royal Library, London. Curiously enough, this drawing is not of Prometheus but of Tityus (fig. 7.10). Prometheus was not the only figure in classical mythology that was punished by having his liver torn out by birds. His fellow Titan Tityus was punished similarly, for the rape of Latona, the mother of Apollo and Artemis. He was banished by Zeus to the Tartarus, , the subterranean realm of the dead in classical antiquity, where he was chained down and visited daily by two vultures that ate parts of his liver. The giant was so large that in his case, two birds were needed to tear out his liver, and yet it still regrew each night. The most significant difference between the stories of Prometheus and Tityus is that Prometheus was chained to the Caucasus Mountains while Tityus was chained in the Tartarus. On the drawing by Michelangelo, the environment doesn't make clear whether we are looking at Tityus or Prometheus, though the bird who acts as torturer is more eagle than vulture. This overlap showcases how difficult it can be to properly delineate between the two myths, and also speaks to the fact that many artists used elements from one myth or the other interchangeably. In this case it's solely through the title of the drawing that Michelangelo makes clear that this is an image of Tityus. The eagle has landed next to Tityus, but hasn't yet made its wound, though the beak is already pointed towards the right side of the chest of the Titan where his liver is located.

Due to the similarities between the two punishments, the composition that Michelangelo used for his Tityus was eagerly adapted for Prometheus depictions by other artists. We see the advent of a new program for the depiction of the body in pain: the pictorial focus shifts from allegorical scenes containing a multitude of figures and episodes to the naked and tortured body itself. Michelangelo thus signifies the development of a new Prometheus type: Prometheus as *torturato*, sufferer. The developing fascination with anatomy and subsequent advances in anatomical study also influenced Renaissance portrayals of the human body. Slowly, the doctrines of Galen were left behind in favour of a more empirical study of the human body.

In this chapter, we have seen how the depiction of scenes from the Prometheus myth developed and changed over the period referred to as the Renaissance. It is clear that primary sources for the myth, found in the works of Hesiodos and Aeschylus, were revisited in order to inform the Renaissance visual program. Elements from these texts that had been left untreated in the Middle Ages found new significance in this period. In the next chapter, we shall discuss the Renaissance knowledge of the liver.

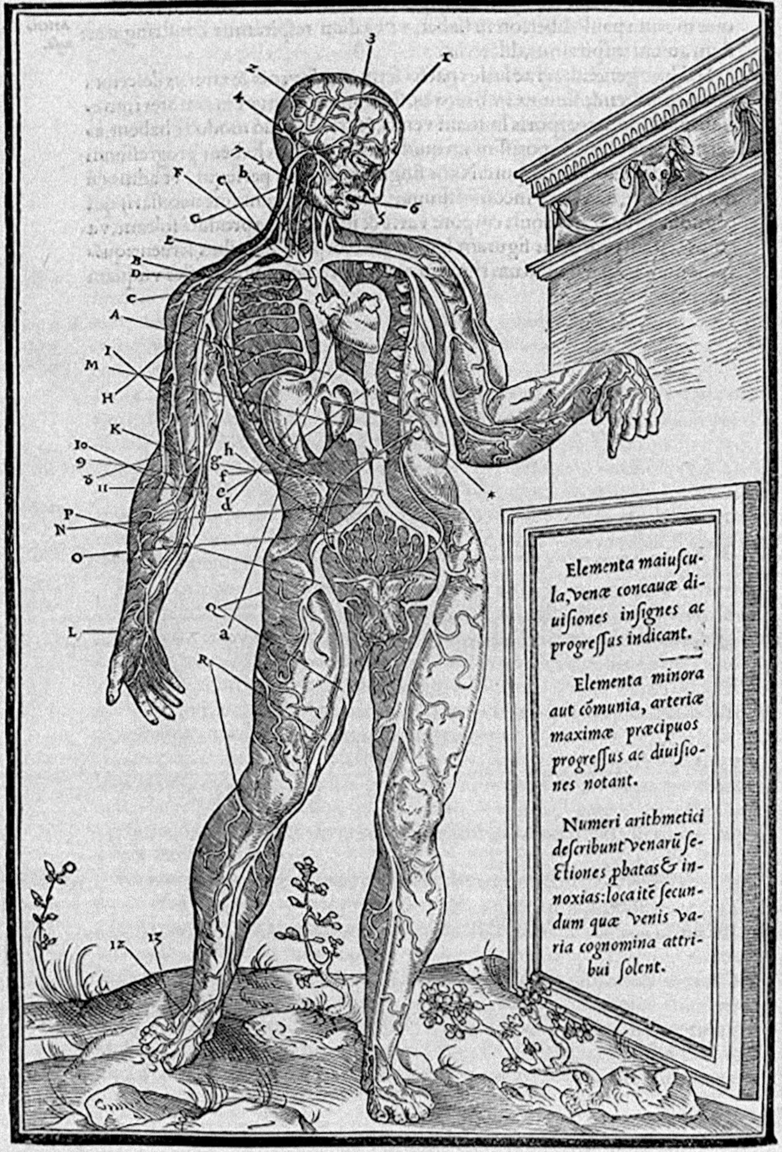
Elementa maiuscu-
la, venæ concauæ di-
uisiones insignes ac
progressus indicant.
Elementa minora
aut cõmunia, arteriæ
maximæ præcipuos
progressus ac diuisio-
nes notant.
Numeri arithmetici
describunt venarũ se-
ctiones ꝓbatas & in-
noxias: loca itẽ secun-
dum quæ venis va-
ria cognomina attri-
bui solent.

8

THE LIVER IN THE RENAISSANCE AS DESCRIBED BY REISCH, VESALIUS, AND DA VINCI

In the beginning of the sixteenth century in Freiburg, somewhere between 1503 and 1519, the Carthusian monk and scholar Gregor Reich published a remarkable work: the *Margarita Philosophica*, which translates to 'the pearl of philosophy.' In this treatise, he outlines the current state of scientific affairs in his era. This voluminous work can be seen as the first encyclopaedia in print, and functions as a scientific conclusion of the Middle Ages forming the base that the Renaissance could be built upon. The book contains a plethora of high-quality, hand-coloured woodcuts to illustrate theories. These include an illustration of the human body showing the positions of the organs in the abdominal cavity (fig. 8.1). As was the case with the few extant medieval anatomical illustrations of this portion of the body, we see a schematic depiction of the liver that shows the organ having multiple lobes. In the upper abdomen and below the diaphragm, we see, from left to right, the liver, the stomach, and the spleen.

The concept of the liver as an organ with five lobes was a continuation of medieval ideas. During this time period, there were very limited opportunities to perform autopsies

Fig. 8.0 The blood-vessels in the human body, including the liver as an organ with multiple lobes in the upper abdominal cavity. Illustration from: De dissectione partium corporis humani libri tres *by Charles Estienne (1504-1564), 1545, Paris*

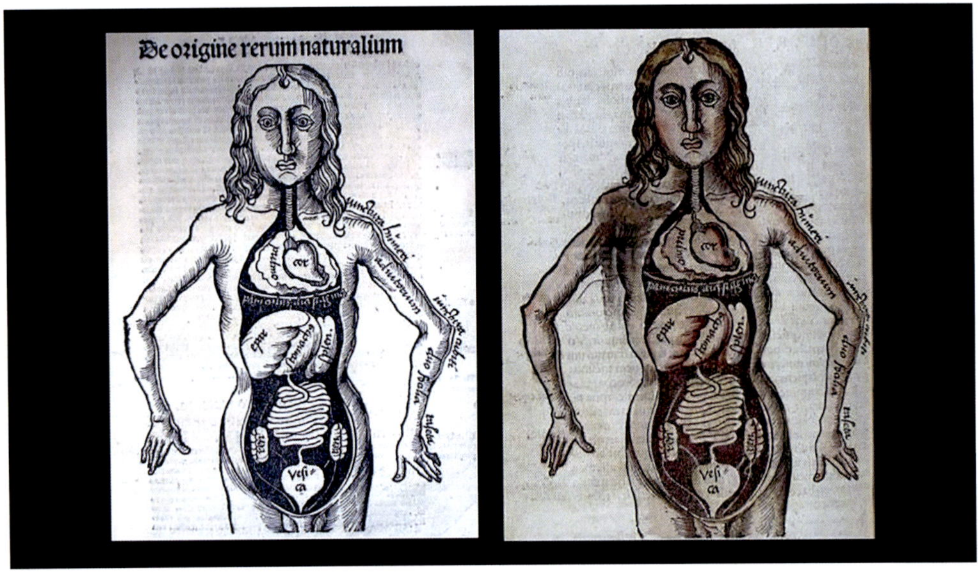

Fig. 8.1 Illustration of the organs in the abdominal cavity, below the diaphragm we see, from left to right, the liver, the stomach and the spleen, from the Margarita Philosophica, *Gregor Reisch (Freiburg 1503)*

on human bodies, which resulted in a rudimentary grasp on the anatomical properties of human organs. The knowledge of the human liver was based entirely on the pig liver, which possesses multiple lobes, in contrast to the human liver, which has two lobes (comparable to that of a sheep, as we have seen in chapter four) (fig. 8.2). It is due to this limited access to the cadaver that, in early Renaissance depictions, the liver is shown as an organ with multiple lobes, following the examples found in pigs.

THE 'FABRICA' OF ANDREAS VESALIUS

One fifteenth-century invention that greatly contributed to the dissemination of anatomical knowledge across Europe was the printing press. The translating, printing, and disseminating of such works by classical scholars like Hippocrates and Galen prompted a

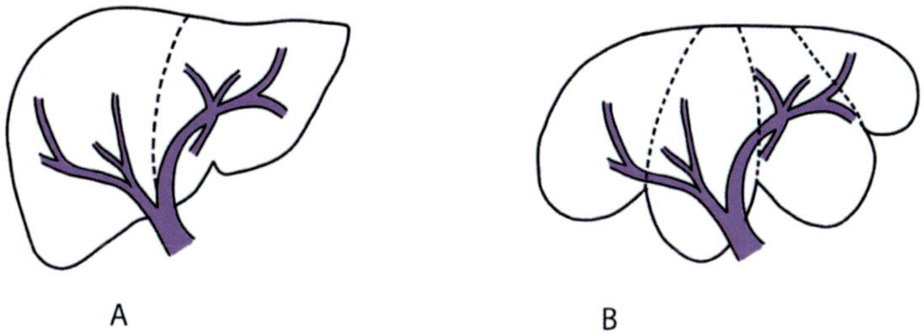

Fig. 8.2 The human liver (left) consists out of two main lobes, while a pig's liver (right) possesses multiple lobes

renewed interest in the ancient Greek healing arts. One of the biggest milestones for the anatomical sciences that the printing press facilitated was the publishing of the first systematic anatomical atlas: *De humani Corporis Fabrica* by Andreas Vesalius (1514-1564). This iconic work formed the basis of a process of self-reinvention within medical sciences, in which the dogmatic doctrines of the Galenic tradition were slowly being let go (fig. 8.3). Once reliant on tradition, society was making way for scientific thought. Vesalius' publication coincided with major reworkings in scientific thought.

Andries van Wesel, who later became known primarily by his latinised name 'Andreas Vesalius,' was born in 1515 in Brussels. His father—stemming from a long lineage of doctors in Wesel in Kleef County—was an apothecary at the court of Maximilian I. After studying philosophy and law at the University of Louvain, Andreas left for Paris, where he studied medicine at the Sorbonne. Conforming to tradition, this institute taught medicine by utilising Galen's teachings. The anatomical education was mainly theoretical in nature and dissections of the human body very rarely took place. Vesalius showed an early interest in anatomy and managed to soon acquire the position of 'prosector' (the person

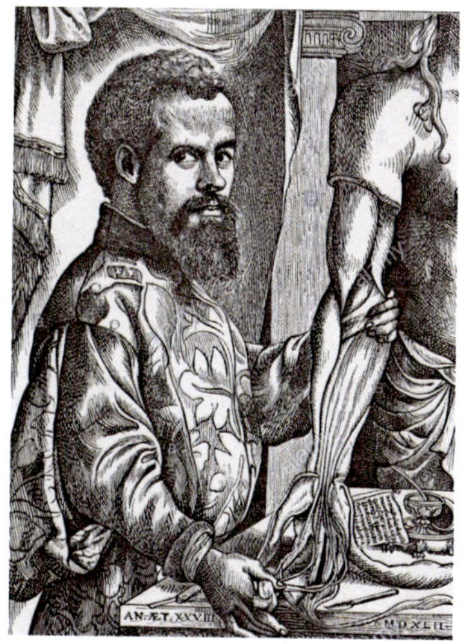

Fig. 8.3 The anatomist Andreas Vesalius (1514-1564) demonstrates the flexor muscles of the lower arm. Author's portrait in De humani corporis fabrica libri septem *(1543)*

Fig 8.4 *Illustration of the liver; the liver is here still depicted as a five lobed organ as can be found in pigs. Andreas Vesalius,* Tabulae anatomicae sex, *Venice (Bernardus Vitalis), 1538. (From: Van Hee 2014, p. 20)*

tasked with performing the dissection on the body) within the faculty. Because of war between France and the Habsburg Empire, Vesalius was forced to leave Paris and return to Louvain to continue his study in medicine. From Louvain he ventured to Padua, where the study of medicine had flourished. He graduated and received his title of medical doctor. In 1537, Vesalius was appointed a professorship in anatomy and surgery at the university of Padua. He taught medicine at the university and utilised the dissection of bodies as an educational tool. During that period, he befriended the artist Jan Stevens van Calcar, who made very detailed drawings of the human skeleton, which Vesalius published in his *Tabulae Anatomica Sex*. This publication also included three images of the circulatory system and the organs. The first of these three depicts the system of the portal vein and the liver—still shown to be a multi-lobbed organ, ever faithful to Galen (fig. 8.4).

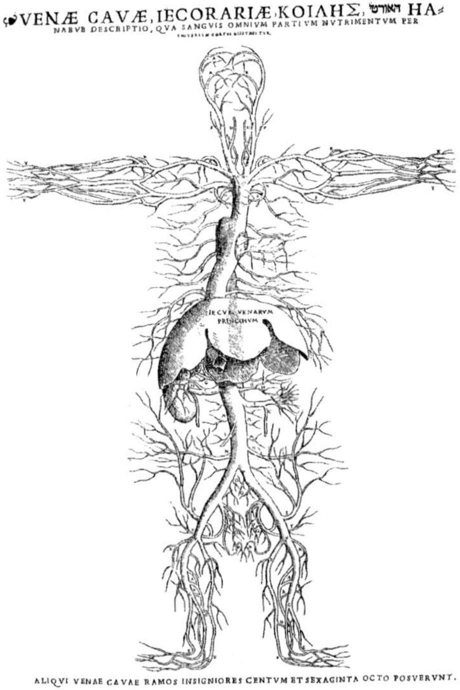

Basing his work on his own empirical observations when dissecting humans, Vesalius began to increasingly question Galen's authority, as the ancient Greek scientist had based his theories mainly on dissections of pigs and other animals. Because of this, when he published his *De Humani Corporis Fabrica Libri Septum* in 1543, he depicted the liver in its true form; that is, as an organ with two lobes (fig. 8.5). This was a controversial image in its time that—along with other critiques of Galen's theory within his publication—brought him massive backlash from established Renaissance anatomists. Despite these criticisms, Vesalius pushed through. For example, in the reprinting of his *Fabrica* from 1555, he depicted the cardiac septum—between the right and left chambers of the heart—as impenetrable, by which he once again opposed centuries of Galenic authority where pores in the cardiac septum were present. The work of Vesalius

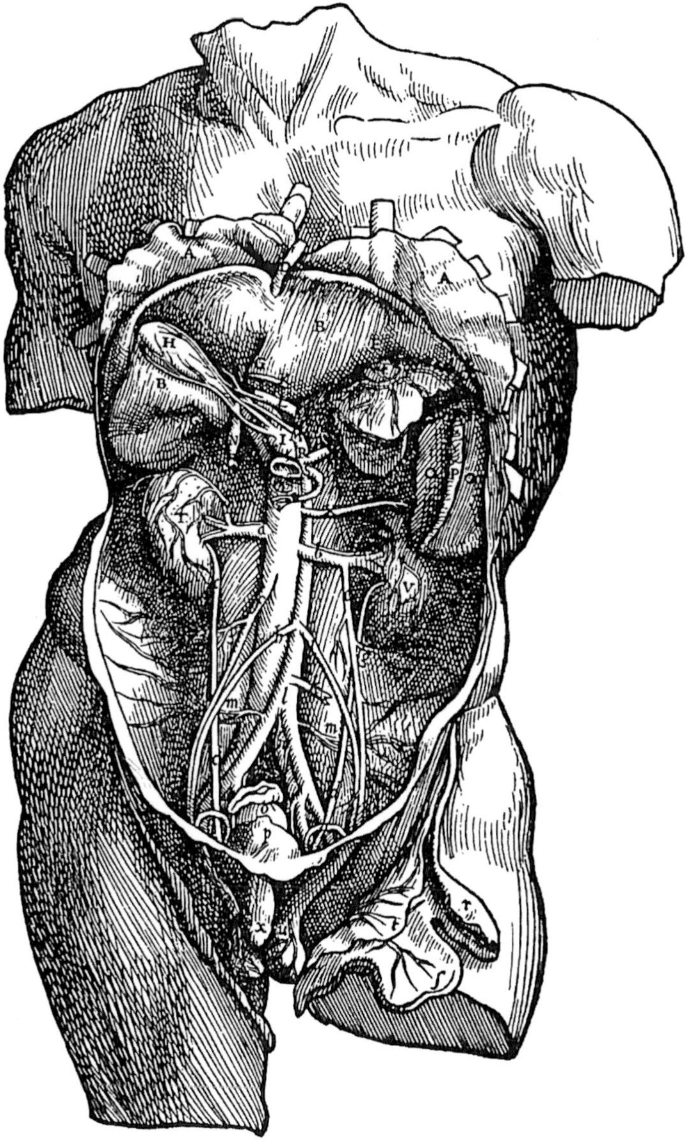

Fig. 8.5 Illustration of the abdominal cavity of a human in Andreas Vesalius, De Humani Corporis Fabrica Libri Septem, *Bazel (Oporinus), 1543, book V, fig. XX (1). In this edition the liver was shown in its true form: as a two lobed organ*

would signify an important turning point in anatomical science, after which a new form of medicinal practice was able to develop.

Of note, in 1545, the anatomical atlas of Charles Estienne (1504-1564) was published: *De Dissectione Partium Corporis Humani Libri Tres*. Together with the surgeon and artist Etienne de la Rivière and the woodcarver Jean Jollat, he produced a series of beautiful and imaginative anatomical plates that were bound together in one book (fig. 8.0). The book was finalised for printing in 1538, but due to a disagreement among the authors the publication was delayed until 1545, two years after the publishing of the *Fabrica* by Vesalius.

In the very same year as Vesalius published his *Fabrica,* Nicolaus Copernicus (1473-1543) published his *theorem* defending the heliocentric model of the universe. This so-called Copernican revolution signified the onset of a radical change in worldview in which the sun, rather than the earth, formed the centre of the universe. Both Vesalius and Copernicus with their groundbreaking visions, contributed to the scientific transformation that evolved at that time.

THE ANATOMICAL NOTES OF LEONARDO DA VINCI

One must also acknowledge the contributions to anatomical science by Leonardo da Vinci, the famed *homo universalis* of the Renaissance, who established himself not only as an artist and inventor, but also as an anatomist. In order to perfect his artistic ability, he sought to gain a thorough understanding of human anatomy in order to depict human bodies in his work in as true to life a manner as possible. As early as 1489, da Vinci produced remarkably accurate drawings of a human skull that he sawed through at different angles in order to examine the inner structure. From da Vinci's notes—which he wrote with his left hand and in a mirrored script—we can understand that he wasn't solely interested in the morphology of the anatomical structure, but that he wanted to understand the development and function of that specific body part as well.

In Florence in 1507, da Vinci performed a dissection on the body of a one hundred-year-old man, in the hope that his organs would reveal the secret of a long life. The man, despite not experiencing any symptoms, turned out to be latently developing a liver disease, which impacted the veins around the liver. Leonardo depicted this condition in the accompanying drawings that he produced for his study (fig. 8.6). To the bottom-left of the drawing, we see the liver in its normal two-lobed form, with the veins, gallbladder and bile duct that connect to the duodenum (depicted as a cross-section). The drawings in the upper-centre and lower-right depict the arteries leading towards the liver, the liver veins culminating in the *vena cava*. These drawings are achieved with a precision unparalleled for the era.

It is clear that da Vinci intended to create an anatomical atlas based on his own drawings and notes, but, due to a variety of circumstances, he was never able to finish the project. He left hundreds of loose folia with anatomical drawings and notes that weren't published until several centuries after his death. After passing between many hands, the collection finally ended up in the possession of the royal family of England, where it was rediscovered in 1773 in the library of Windsor Castle. The entire collection of anatomical drawings and notes by da Vinci was published as a facsimile edition in 1898. Had his anatomical work been discovered earlier, da Vinci may have been canonised as *the* anatomical reformer of the Renaissance.

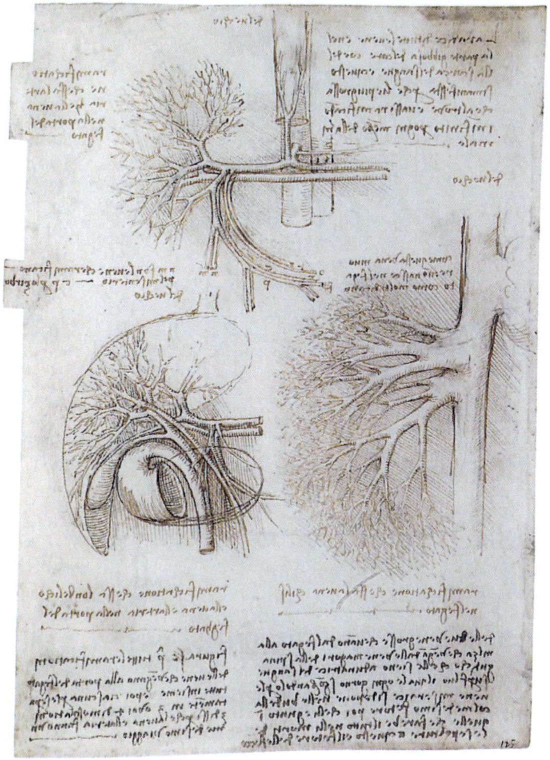

Fig. 8.6 Leonardo da Vinci, Drawings of the blood vessels around the liver, made during a dissection of a deceased hundred-year-old man. To the bottom left we see the two lobed liver with the gallbladder and a bile duct leading to the (cross-sectioned) duodenum. 1507, (From: Clayton en Philo 2017, p. 95)

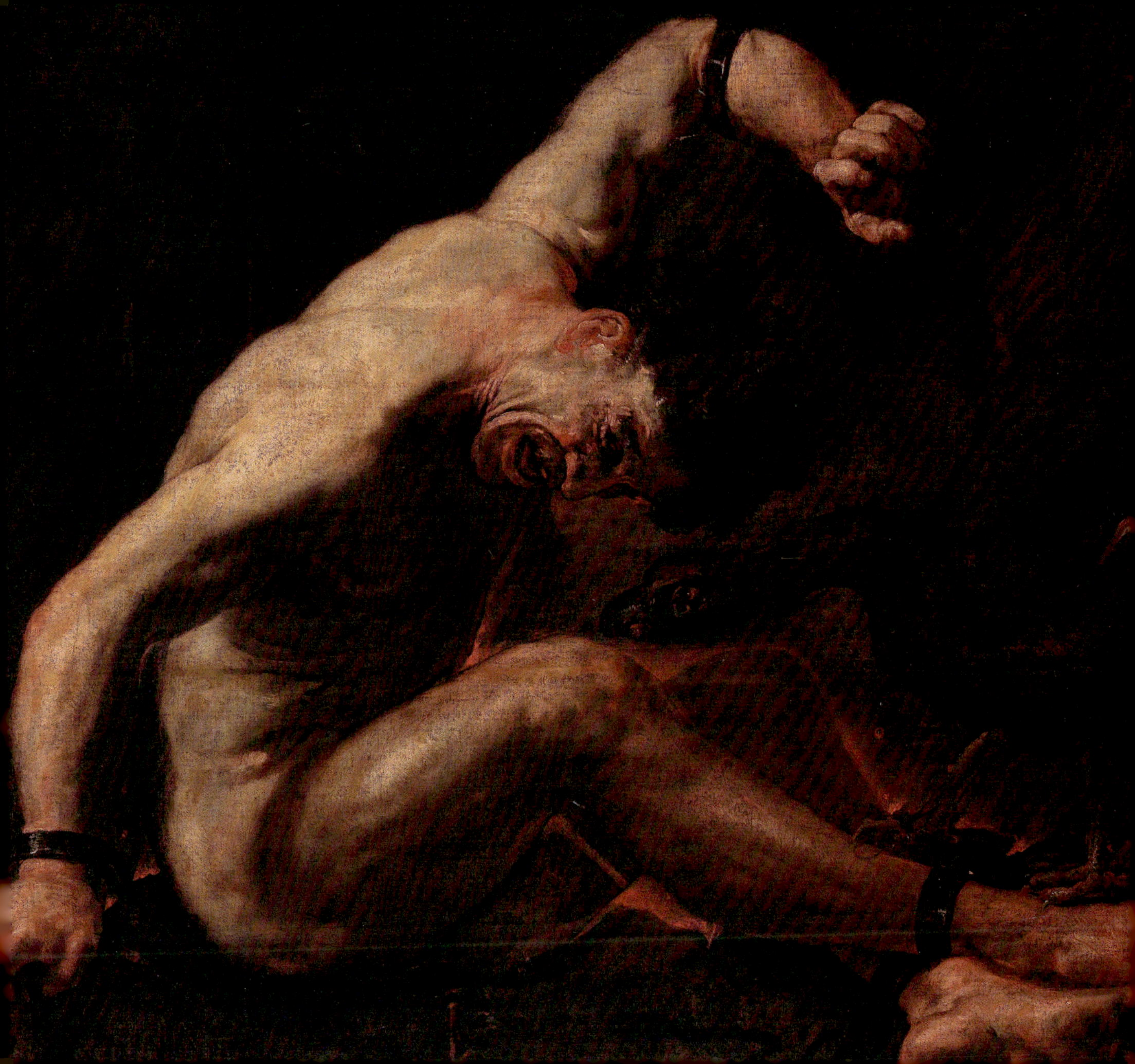

9

PROMETHEUS IN THE BAROQUE

During the transition from the Renaissance to the Baroque, we see a shift in the way Prometheus is depicted: he changes from heroic thinker to heroic tortured nude. In this chapter, we will showcase the masterpieces of this era that take up Prometheus as their subject, and consider why the punishment of Prometheus formed the ideal motif through which artists expressed seventeenth-century artistic sensibilities.

Fig. 9.0 Assereto Gioacchino, the punishment of Prometheus, oil on canvas, 1620-1649, 119 × 155 cm, Colnaghi gallery, London

The term 'baroque' may come from the Portuguese word 'barroco', which means 'flawed pearl'. Even though the transition from the Renaissance to the Baroque is a gradual one, the increase in drama and caprice in the manner of depiction that we witness from the sixteenth to seventeenth centuries speaks to the arrival of a new and distinct artistic style. This transition is often compared to the key development in the ancient Greek art, where we see a shift from the serene 'Classical' period to the dramatic 'Hellenistic' one. In the Renaissance, the classical past was met with a new appreciation, and the art of the 'Classical' period was deemed ideal. The balance of bodily proportions and the often-symmetrical composition were thought to contain a serenity that should be pursued, while the more emotional Hellenistic art was seen as a disturbance and degeneration of this delicate balance.

Fig. 9.1 Titian, Tityus chained in the Tartarus, while the eagle eats his liver. c. 1565. Oil paint on canvas, 253 x 217 cm. Museo Nacional del Prado, Madrid

In the Renaissance, the depiction of emotions was often restricted to expression on the face. This was especially true in the mannerism of the High Renaissance (roughly 1490-1527), which was characterised by strict formulaic norms. The artists of the Baroque, however, shook of this formulaic yoke and found an appreciation for Hellenistic art, in which the body functioned as a canvas for the soul. Emotions were no longer solely expressed on the face, but within the entire body, from the twisted face to the curled toes.

A second characteristic of Baroque art can be revealed with a remark that Michelangelo (1475-1564) made concerning the work of the Venetian painter Titian (1490-1576). He complained that the latter didn't posses enough *disegno* in his work—that is to say, a command of linework and design. Titian worked more with colour and light – a method that would greatly gain popularity in the North during the Dutch Golden Age of painting (about 1588 to 1672). The difference between the styles was determined by how 'true to life' ('naer het leven' or 'ad vivum') artwork seemed to be; northern painters were known to include all the small details in their works, highlighting blemishes and impurities. Within the aesthetic boundaries of the *disegno* of the Renaissance, there were certain properties of the visible world that could be depicted and others that could not. In order to achieve idealised beauty, only that which was designated beautiful could be memorialised in paint. The *disegno* of the Italian renaissance used the golden mean of the human body as an anchoring point. Everything that would cause one to zoom out too far and only depict humans as small figurines, nor everything that would cause one to zoom in too far and depict all small details that would only be noticeable when one looked through a lens, was not considered fit for depiction. The artists of the Italian renaissance often leveraged this preference as a critique of different cultures, especially of their northern colleagues, where these macroscopic and microscopic modes of depiction were more prevalent.

TITYUS AS A PROMETHEAN PROTOTYPE

One of the biggest influences on the depiction of Prometheus in the Baroque is found in a painting of a different Titan: the Tityus, by Titian. In this work, the artist took the

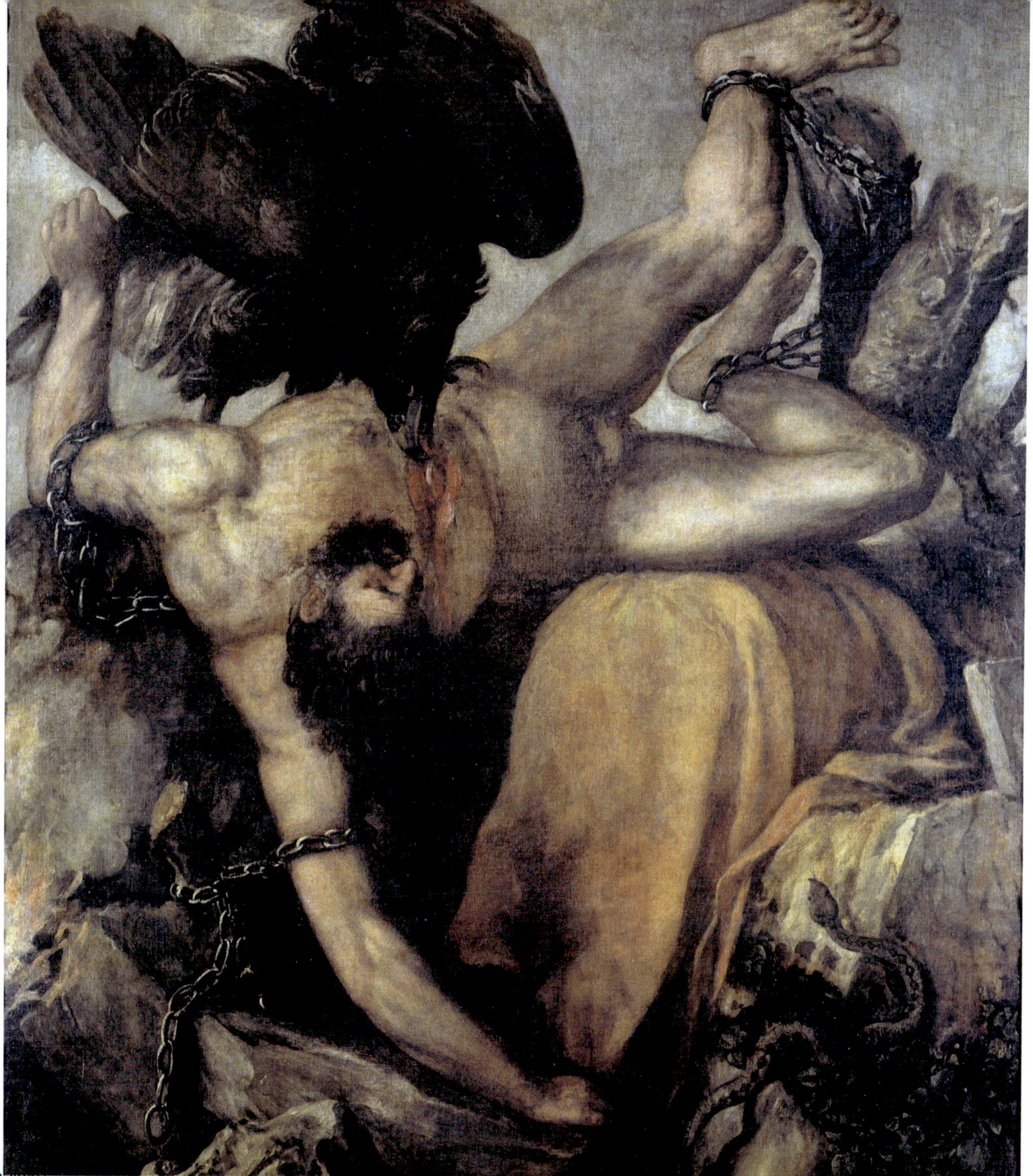

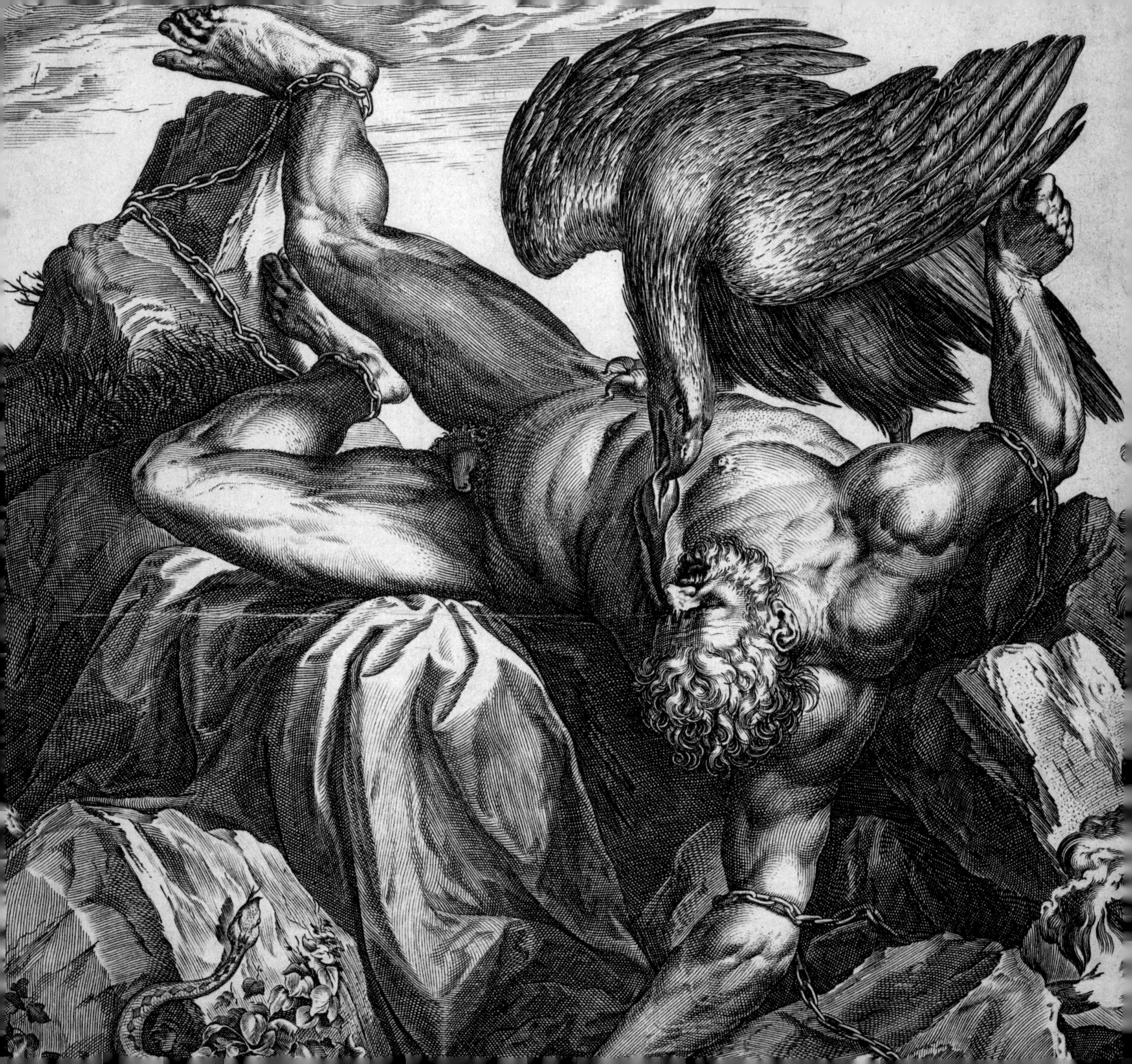

drawing of Tityus by Michelangelo from 1533 (fig. 7.10) – as discussed in chapter 7 – as his starting point. He then proceeded to, as it were, tip Tityus backwards, changing the horizontal composition into a diagonal one. The rocks below Tityus' head are lower than those at his feet, a visual paradox that creates a dramatic and almost precarious pivot. Titian's first iteration of this work has, unfortunately, been lost. Thankfully, we can still get a decent idea of what it might have looked like thanks to the copy he made of the work, which is now displayed at the Prado in Madrid (fig. 9.1). A second copy of Titian's original, Cornelis Cort's (1533-1578) engraving of the image gives further insight into the Promethean visual program (fig. 9.2). Cort made several key changes to Titian's composition. One difference is that the composition is flipped: when engravings are printed onto paper, this results in a mirroring of the image, unless the etching on the engraving plate has been completed backwards. Another change Cort made was to the location the sufferer is tortured in: instead of in a dark underworld, the Titan now lies in the open air, and, in the lower-right corner, a burning torch sticks out between two shards of rock. This points to a change of identity in Cort's engraving, which is confirmed in the subscript of the image. Cort has depicted Prometheus, where Titian had made Tityus his subject. Thanks to the reproducible nature of the medium, the dissemination of Cort's engraving simultaneously produced the dissemination of the myth and visual program of Prometheus.

Fig. 9.2 Cornelis Cort after Titian, Prometheus chained to the rocks of the Caucasus, 1566. engraving, 368 x 312 mm. Rijksmuseum, Amsterdam

RUBENS SETS THE BAR HIGH

Cort's engraving also reached Peter Paul Rubens (1577-1640), one of the most famous artists of the Southern Netherlands, who, in 1612, gave the Promethean subject his own spin (fig. 9.3). Dominicus Baudius (1561-1633), the artist's contemporary and admirer, praised Rubens' painting of Prometheus. Baudius wrote that the tortured Prometheus gave off the impression that, were he not restrained by his chains, he would topple backwards out of the painting and land on the spectator. The poet also allots a large portion of his praise to the eagle, even though he erroneously calls it a vulture – clearly confusing this element from the myth of Tityus, whose liver was torn out by two vultures instead

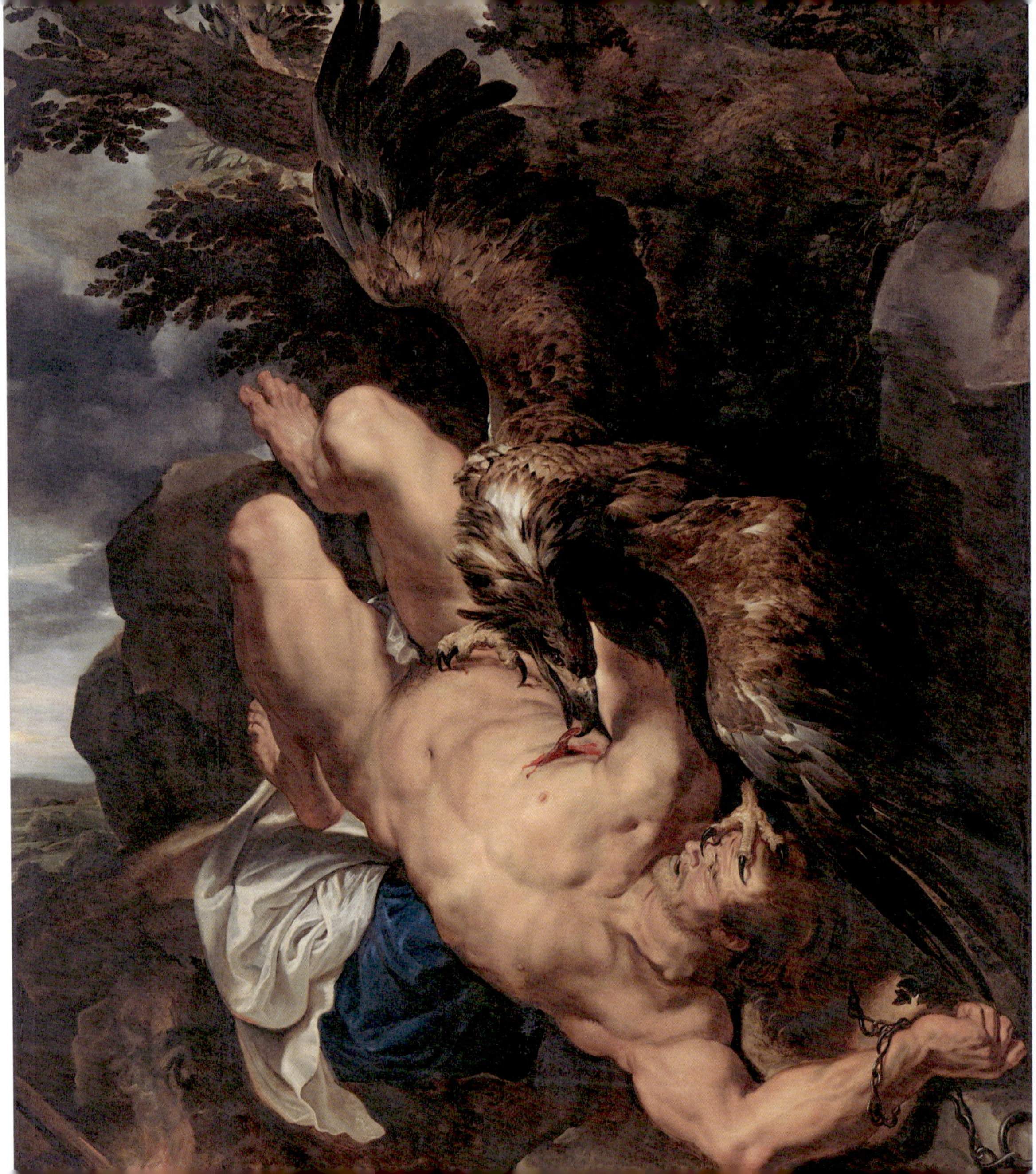

of the sole eagle. He wrote that the wind caused by the large wings of the bird was nearly felt on the face of the spectator, and that the bird's eyes were alight with flames.

Rubens depicted Prometheus on this canvas – now in the Philadelphia Museum of Art – as a heroic nude. He positioned the figure in a strong diagonal in the composition, his feet in the upper-left corner and the head in the lower-right. The diagonal of the figure is mirrored by both the wings of the eagle and the foliage and branches of the tree behind them. The eagle doesn't just have in his beak Prometheus' torn-away skin; he has also cruelly planted his claws in the Titan's thigh and face. While Baudius lauded the eagle as the work of Rubens, it was not actually painted by him. From the artist's correspondences, we know that the eagle was painted by Frans Snyders (1579-1657), a famous painter of both living birds and hunted fowl. Snyders' pencil study for this painting survives and is held in the collection of the British Museum, further corroborating this collaboration between Rubens and Snyders. (fig. 9.4).

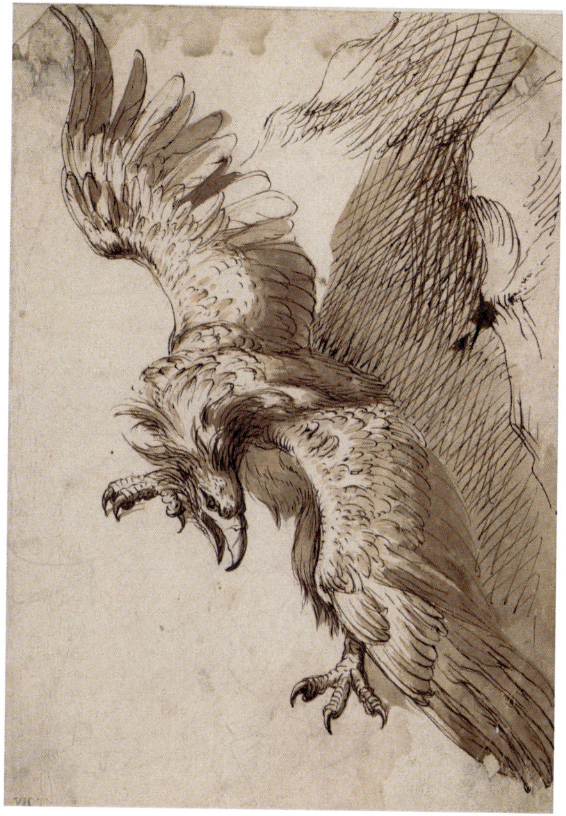

Fig. 9.3 Peter Paul Rubens, the punishment of Prometheus. The eagle has dug his claws into the face and the leg of Prometheus. It has part of his liver, that it has torn out of a wound in the right side of his chest, in its beak. In the lower left corner, we see the torch that Prometheus used to carry the fire to the humans. 1611-1612, oil paint on canvas, 244 x 210 cm, Philadelphia Museum of Art, Philadelphia

Fig. 9.4 Frans Snyders. Study for the eagle of Prometheus, c. 1610. Pen drawing in brown ink, 280 x 202 mm. British Museum, London

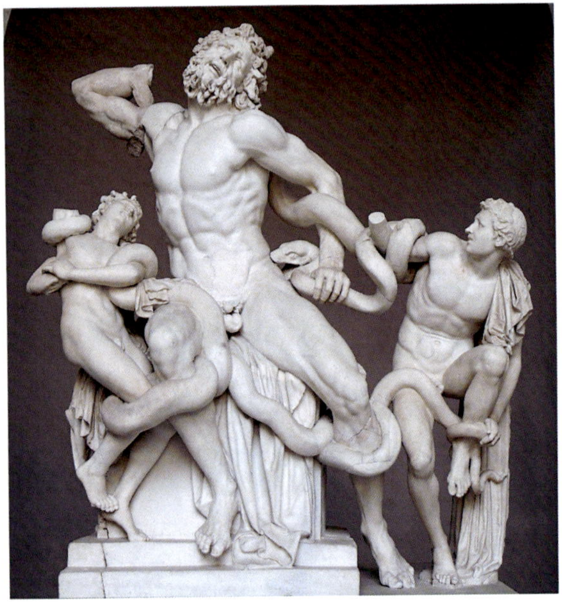

THE IMITATION OF ANTIQUITY

Rubens depicts Prometheus with one knee pulled up and the other leg outstretched – a pose we see most commonly in Rubens' oeuvre in his depictions of someone in great suffering. He seems to have emulated this formula from antique examples. It is known that Rubens made studies of one of the most famous Hellenistic statue groups: the marble Laocoön group, excavated in 1506 in Rome (fig. 9.5). It depicts the priest Laocoön and his sons as they are being strangled and bitten by snakes. The marble sculptors have depicted suffering of and in the body: the figures in pain lift one knee up while stretching out their other leg to express great stress on the body. Rubens did not only copy the pose of the legs for his Prometheus; he also made a study of the priest's muscular torso, emulating the figure's prominent ribs and broad chest as the basis for the torso of his Prometheus.

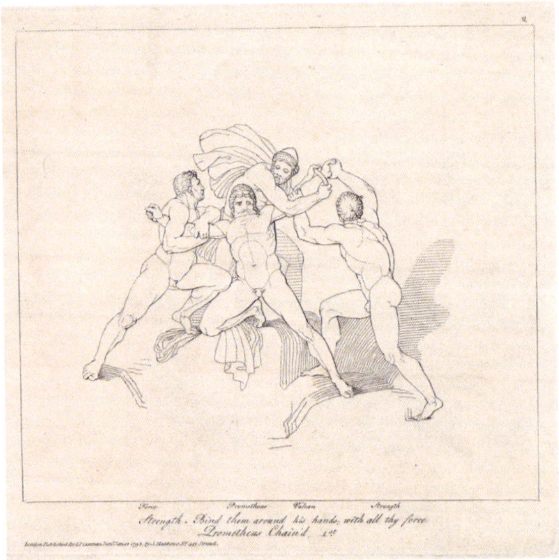
Force
Prometheus
Vulcan
Strength
Strength. Bind them around his hands, with all thy force
Prometheus Chain'd, 1st

Fig. 9.5 Laocoön group. The Trojan priest Laocoön and his two sons are being strangled by serpents sent by the sea god Poseidon for trying to prevent that the Trojan horse would be brought into the city. White marble, 27 CE, attributed to Hagesander, Polydorus and Athenodoros of Rodos, unearthed in 1506 in a vineyard in Rome, Vatican Museum, Rome.

Fig. 9.6 Tommaso Piroli after John Flaxman, Prometheus chained to the rock by Hephaistos (the smith of the gods), Cratus (power), and Bia (Violence). Engraving for an edition of the tragedy by Aeschylus, 1795, 176 x 200 mm, Royal Academy of Arts, London

The connection between Prometheus and Laocoön as exemplars of heroic suffering is drawn even more explicitly by Giovanni Paolo Lomazzo (1538-1592). In his *Trattato dell'arte della pitura*, written in 1585, Lomazzo writes that after grief, pain was the most powerful passion to portray in art because pain influences the entire body. He mentions Prometheus and Laocoön as subjects in whom such suffering can be best depicted. Laocoön developed into the icon of pain in western art. This comparison is perfectly illustrated in an engraving by Tommaso Piroli (1752-1824) after a drawing by John Flaxman (1755-1826) from 1795, despite the later date of the drawing. Here, the comparison between Prometheus and Laocoön is taken literally, as he portrays the Titan in the exact same position as the priest.

PROMETHEUS BY JORDAENS: FARCICAL OR A DIVINE COMEDY?

Rubens' painting, *Prometheus Bound*, was widely influential, a designation that becomes apparent when we compare it with a painting by Jacob Jordaens (1593-1678) from 1640 with the same title (fig. 9.7). The two works show many similarities, —the eagle is completely identical—making it hard to tell the two works apart. However, there are several important differences between the compositions. Jordaens has forgone the strong diagonal composition that Rubens used in favour of a more upright position, placing the Titan on the left half of the canvas and thus freeing up space for additional figures at the right. In addition to the burning torch – the necessary attribute to identify Prometheus – Jordaens also depicts other elements from the myth. Hermes is present, placed behind the tree Prometheus is bound to, looking at the chained Titan with a gloating smile. Between the rocks, we see a sculpture of a woman and a piece of glistening fat-covered bones. Prometheus' disposition is different as well, when compared to Rubens' figure; where Rubens depicts Prometheus undergoing his torture with a stoic dignity, Jordaens shows him wailing with a wide-open mouth and wild eyes. In the early modern perception such displays of emotion were in opposition with intelligence.

For a long time, the perceived lack of dignity present in Jordaens' suffering Prometheus was attributed to the fact that the painter worked for a bourgeois patronage rather than

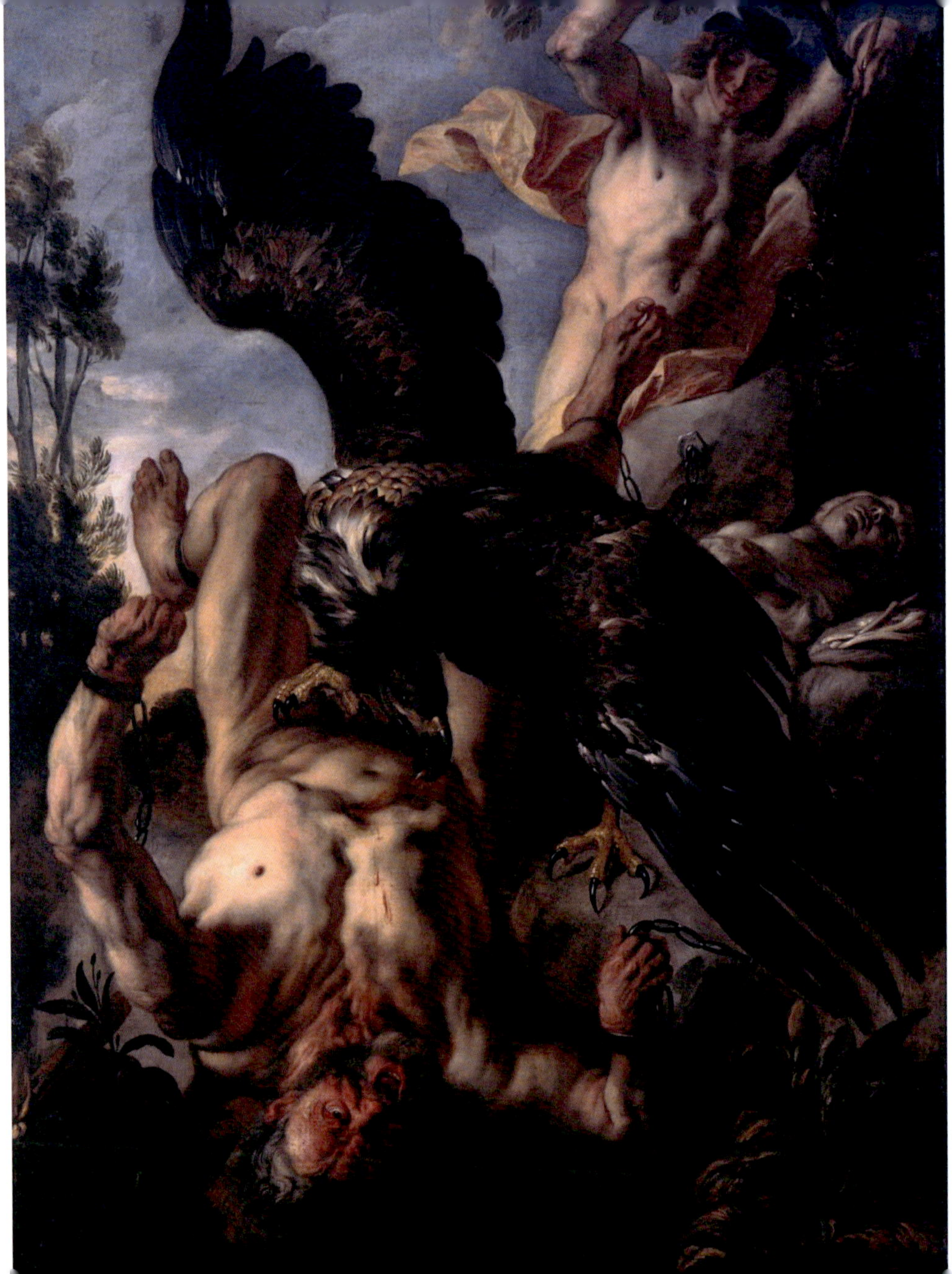

Fig. 9.7 Jacob Jordaens, The punishment of Prometheus. Prometheus was punished for a threefold crime: deceiving Zeus during the sacrifice at mecone, creating humans, and stealing the fire. Jordaens drew on the comedy by Lucianus for his composition. c. 1640, oil paint on canvas, 245 x 178 cm, Walraff-Richartz Museum, Cologne

a noble one, and that he was mainly interested in running a profit, which would explain the lack of intellectual gravitas. Recent studies, however, have proposed that it is possible that Jordaens used a different textual source for his painting, which would account for the differences between his work and Rubens' without dismissing the Jordaens' intellect or audience.

The comedic version of the myth of Prometheus by Lucian of Samosata (died 192 CE) is the only text that unites all of the elements depicted in Jordaens' painting. In both Lucian's version and Aeschylus' version, Hephaistus, the divine smith, was responsible for chaining Prometheus to the mountain, but in Lucian's text, Hermes appointed the location of the Titan's punishment. While Prometheus undergoes his punishment with a taciturn dignity in Aeschylus, in Lucian's work, he bemoans his fate and complains that the punishment is unjustified. Hermes explains to him that he is being punished for three crimes: the deceit with the sacrificial meat, the creation of humans, and the theft of the fire, as described in the first chapter. Prometheus objects to each of these accusations. He argues each point: surely Zeus wasn't so petty that he'd complain over finding a little bone left in his stew; and that, if Zeus really was so upset about his creation of humans, he spent a remarkable amount of time sleeping with mortal women; and finally, that since the humans had obtained fire, the gods did not have less fire, as the element multiplies itself. Each of these were valid counterarguments, but Lucian lets Hermes have the last word. Hermes sarcastically tells Prometheus that he hopes he'll still come to dinner parties on Olympus, so long as he's not the one bringing the meat.

It's probably this last statement by Hermes that Jordaens intended to depict. The three attributes (the torch, the sacrificial meat, and the statue) represent the three crimes that Prometheus was punished for. The text by Lucian is the only text that contains both the three attributes as well as the presence of a laughing and sarcastic Hermes. Lucian's comedy has remained unnoticed as a possible source for a long time because only the more serious works by Hesiod and Aeschylus were really considered. In short, we should pause before unduly accusing Jordaens of lacking intellectual gravitas, when he did likely

Afb. 9.8 Prometheus wordt in de ketenen geslagen door Hephaistos, terwijl Hermes lachend toekijkt. Op de voorgrond zien we instrumenten en op de achtergrond scènes uit de Tartarus, zoals de vork van Hades en Ixion op het rad gebonden. De adelaar (linksboven) wacht geduldig tot de goden klaar zijn met het ketenen van de titaan. Dirck van Baburen, 1623 Olieverf op doek, 202 x 184 cm, Rijksmuseum, Amsterdam

base his work on a comedic antique text. His less severe treatment of the subject is better suited to the comical nature of the text by Lucian.

A second reason to think that it was probably Lucian's text that Jordaens based his work on is the widespread popularity of this author in both the Northern and the Southern Netherlands. Lucian's work was translated from the less accessible Greek to the more common Latin and then into the French vernacular. Additionally, Lucian was an author often read by artists because he gave descriptions of the lost works of legendary painters from ancient Greece, like Apelles. Following these descriptions, Baroque artists would try to reconstruct and emulate these ancient painters solely by closely following these texts.

VAN BABUREN'S PROMETHEUS IN THE TARTARUS

The Prometheus painted by Dirck van Baburen (1595-1624) was also likely based on the text by Lucian (fig. 9.8). Just like with Jordaens, we once again see some visual comparisons with the work by Rubens; here, the *topos* of the stretched leg and one pulled up knee to signify suffering was used as well. This painting was also subjected to harsh judgement for its supposed 'low' style. The ruddy face of Prometheus and the gleeful smirk of Hermes were deemed even more farcical than in the work by Jordaens. In a certain sense, van Baburen stayed more faithful to Lucian's text by depicting both Hermes and Hephaistus. In van Baburen's work, Prometheus is yet to be tortured by the eagle, which is patiently waiting for him behind Hephaistus, who is in the act of chaining Prometheus. The attributes of the crimes that Prometheus is being punished for are harder to identify in this painting. Instead of a torch, we see a compass, protractor, and books—a possible reference to all the different types of knowledge (mathematics, astronomy, etc.) that humanity could develop after Prometheus brought them the fire.

A remarkable departure from the story as told by Lucian in van Baburen's work is that the artist's version doesn't seem to be situated on the Caucasus Mountains but deep within Tartarus: the ancient Greek underworld. At first glance, the fiery glow would suggest

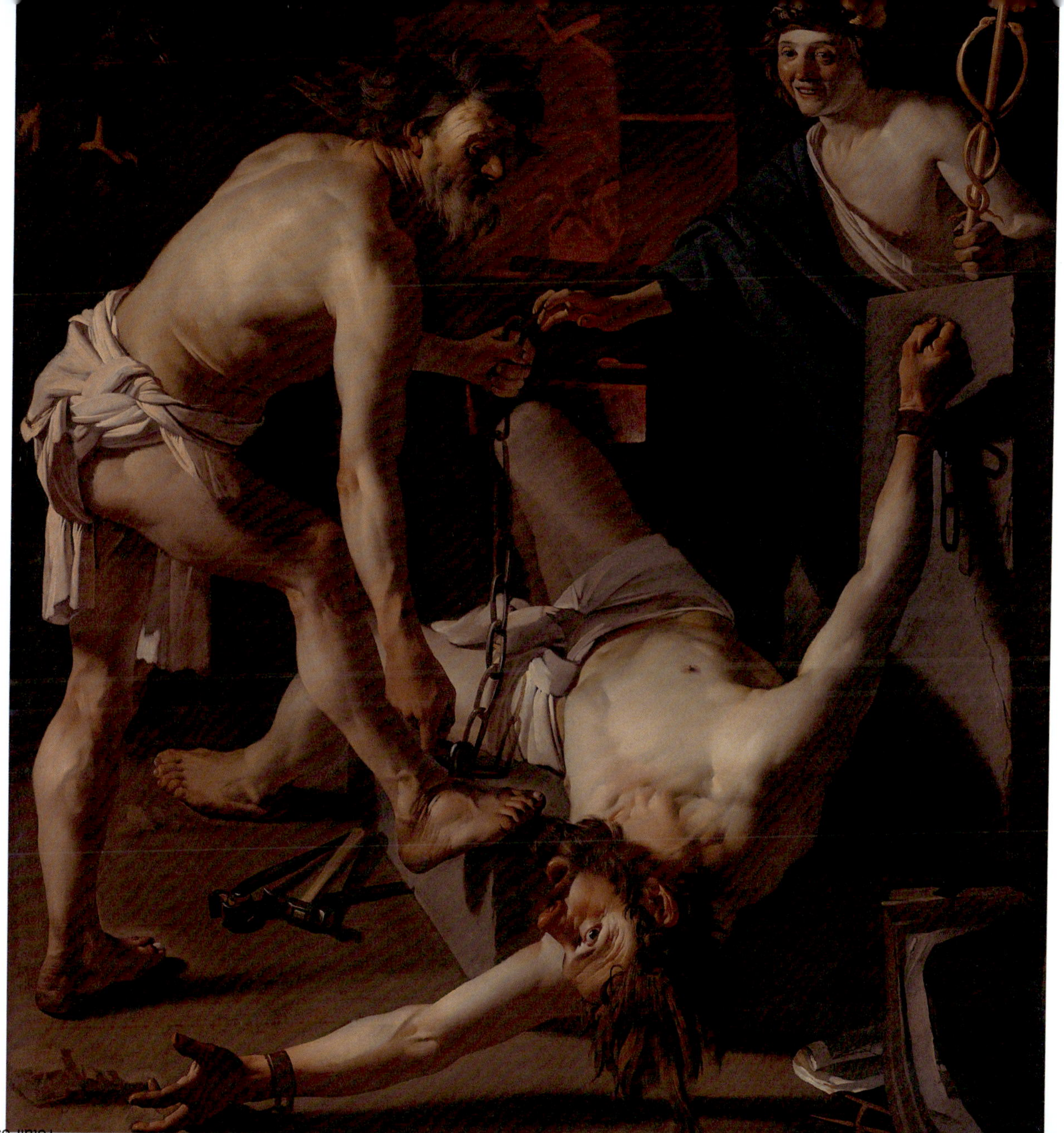

that this is merely the workplace of Hephaistus, but when we look through the small window, we can see a two-pronged pitchfork – which was the attribute of Hades – and in the sea of flames, we see someone who is bound to a spinning wheel. This would be Ixion, a king who was punished by Zeus for attempting to seduce Hera. He was punished by being tied to a flaming wheel that would turn for all eternity in Tartarus. It is clear that a certain confusion concerning the subject matter has also crept into the painting by van Baburen, as the two iconographies have become strongly intertwined—are we looking at Prometheus or is this Tityus?

SALVATOR ROSA AND THE SUBLIME SCREAM OF PROMETHEUS

As is shown by the many pieces of seventeenth-century art that make Prometheus' muscular naked torso the central focus, the art of that era is characterised by a heightened interest in a realistic portrayal of the body. This interest in the body went hand in hand with a development in scientific thought during the so-called 'scientific revolution'. In the Renaissance the established scientific presence still preferred to rely on tradition and handed-down wisdom– with the exception of a few visionaries. During the course of the seventeenth century, this type of knowledge was increasingly replaced with an attention to empiricism and experiment, including the performing of dissections in order to gain insight into human anatomy. These dissections were often witnessed by artists who wished to improve their grasp on depicting human anatomy in a way that was true to nature and as we have seen in the case of Leonardo da Vinci, sometimes even performed by them.

A second important societal development that influenced art in the seventeenth century was the schism between the Catholic and Protestant Church and the wars of religion prompted by it. In response to the growing popularity of Protestantism, the Catholic Church had to re-profile itself in order to re-establish its appeal in the face of such harsh criticism. In the art world, this led to, among other things, the art of the Catholic Counterreformation. Counterreformation art was characterised by a heightened presence of emotion and an immersive character in order to inspire deep religious experience in viewers, thus providing something that the aniconic and iconoclastic Protestant Church could not offer.

Within this movement, there emerged a new fascination with the notion of the 'sublime,' a concept that was first defined by the ancient philosopher Longinus. The 'sublime' was a specific subtype of aesthetic experience that could be brought on to someone by witnessing something, either in art or in nature, that fit certain characteristics. The sublime wasn't necessarily beautiful, but rather an awe-inspiring state in which all words fail. An overwhelming thunderstorm or the violence of a turbulent ocean or the eruption of a volcano were often given as examples of the sublime. Simultaneous advancements in science brought parts of nature to light that had been previously unknown or unexplored. The magnificent scale and changeability of this newly discovered world touched upon this feeling evoked by the sublime. According to Jesuit thinkers of the Counterreformation, the magnitude of God could be felt in this sublime experience of nature through science.

Salvator Rosa (1615-1673), an Italian painter who worked at the papal court of the Barberini utilised the concept of the sublime in his art. The Barberini court encouraged an environment where these ideals and philosophies of the Counterreformation were especially prevalent. For his debut as a painter in Rome, Rosa painted Prometheus being besieged by the eagle (fig. 9.9). In this painting (completed between 1646 and 1648), we see the new fascination for the anatomical joined with the overwhelming force of the sublime. Prometheus is depicted lying down, chained to the rocks of the Caucasus Mountains. While Rubens and Jordaens have the eagle pull out the liver through a relatively small wound, Salvator Rosa has the bird tear open Prometheus' stomach to such an extent that his organs are slipping out of his stomach cavity. In his upturned beak, the eagle holds a part of Prometheus' large intestine, while the liver lies dark and glistening in the Titan's own lap. Prometheus almost functions here as a dramatized anatomical lesson, a genre popularised in Netherlandish art.

The sublime drama that Rosa managed to capture in his painting was widely praised by his contemporaries. Paolo Vendramin, the Venetian ambassador in Florence and a

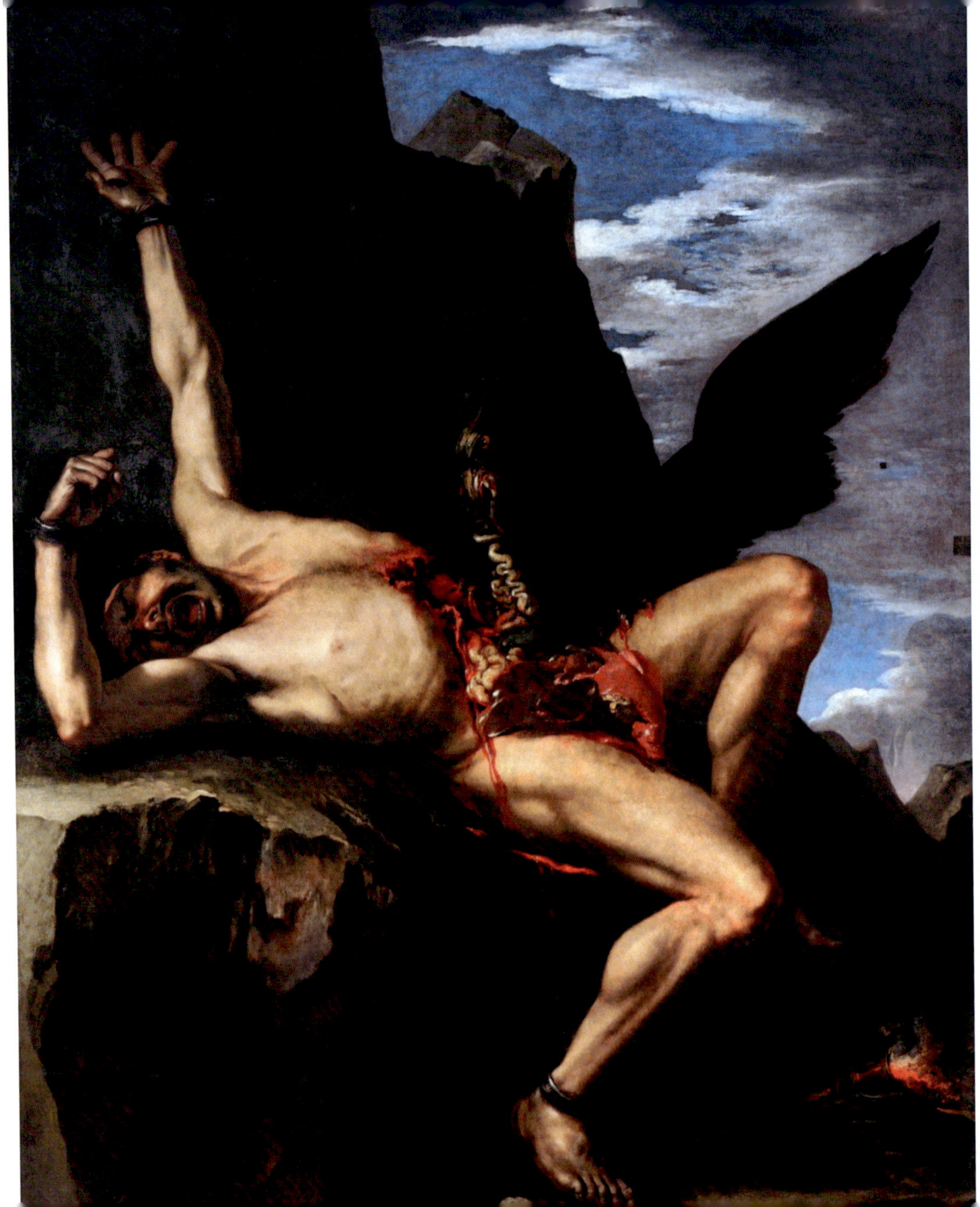

contemporary of Rosa, compared Rosa's Prometheus with lightning painted by the legendary painter of antiquity, Apelles. According to legend (all works by Apelles have been lost), Apelles had managed to depict that which cannot be depicted. Supposedly, lightning was so bright that it wasn't paintable. Instead, he painted the darkened contours of the hand of Zeus holding the lightning, thus suggesting the lightning through contrast and negative space. The sublime is reserved exactly for these types of magnitudes that suspend understanding, painting what cannot be painted . Vendramin saw a similar principle in the voiceless scream of Prometheus painted by Rosa. The scream was so intense that, according to Vendramin, the spectator could feel the mortal peril that Prometheus was in—this peril was so grand that it could only be felt, rather than depicted. Vendramin proclaimed Rosa as a visionary, as the artist managed to capture a cry – something belonging to the auditory and not the visual – in the visual realm, and made it almost audible through his painting. In short, Rosa made Prometheus' pain tangible.

Fig. 9.9 Salvator Rosa, The punishment of Prometheus. Prometheus is chained to the Caucasus. The eagle has torn open his abdomen and a large part of his organs have spilled into his lap. 1646-1648, oil paint on canvas, 224 × 179 cm, Galleria Nazionale d'Arte Antica in Palazzo Corsini, Rome

In this chapter, we have seen how, in the seventeenth century, Prometheus was turned into a martyr of heroic suffering, a subject made the central focus of many a monumental painting. His noble suffering sometimes took on Christ-like dimensions. The fascination with the body in pain and the desire to depict bodies in as realistic a manner as possible—with great attention to anatomical correctness—went hand in hand with developments in medical science. These developments and their relationship to art will be elaborated upon in the next chapter.

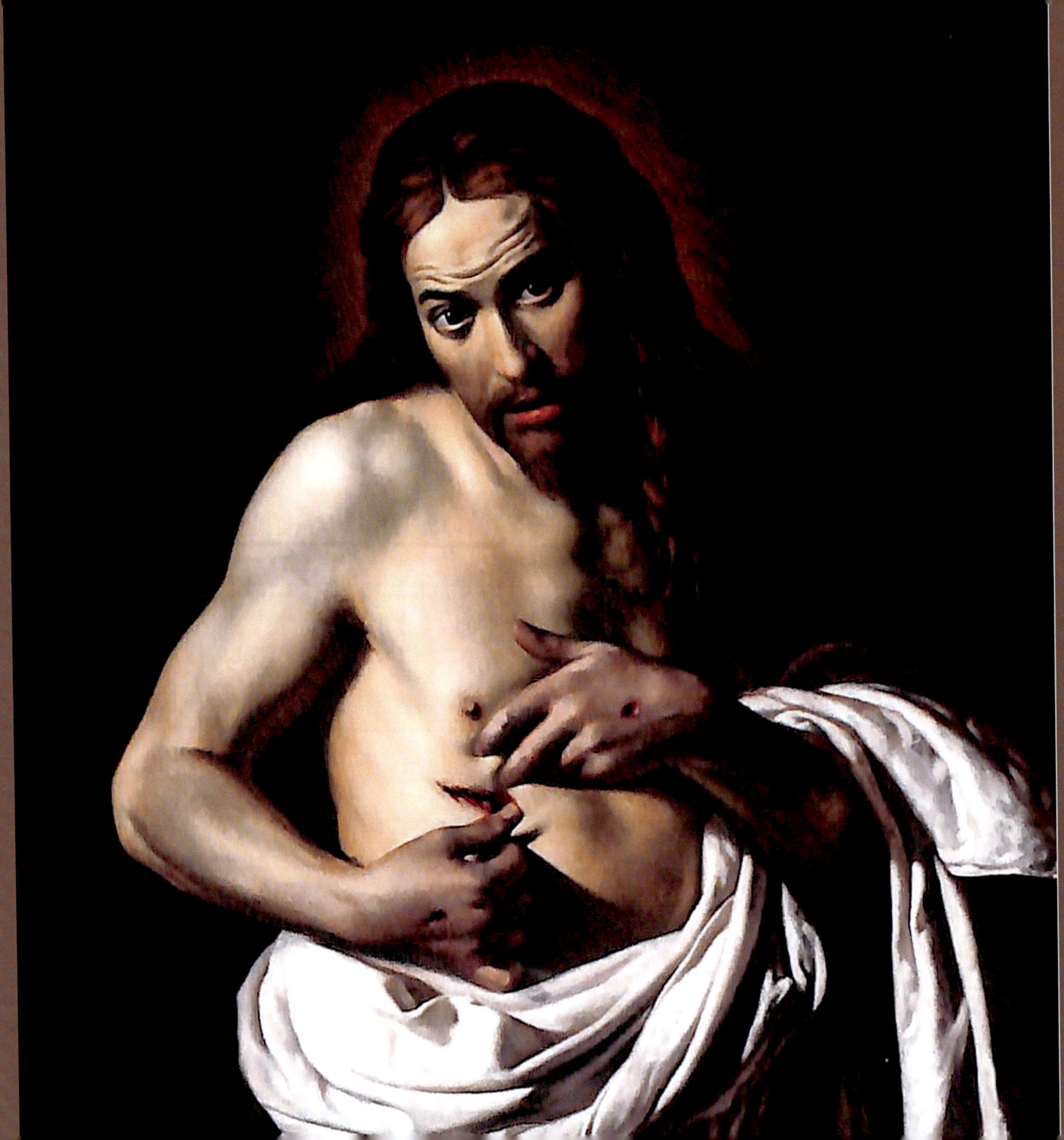

THE WOUNDS OF CHRIST AND PROMETHEUS – TWO OF A KIND?

It isn't hard to see how Prometheus and Christ might register as thematically similar. Both brought selfless and personal sacrifices to the benefit of humanity, accomplished through intense bodily suffering. In the chapter on the depiction of Prometheus in the Baroque, we covered the seventeenth-century fascination for naturalistic depictions of the human body, paired with a fondness for depicting drama and pathos. Bodily suffering aptly combined these two trends. Both the Passion of Christ and the punishment of Prometheus are subject matters that allow for this much sought-after combination of anatomy and pathos. The visual correspondence between Prometheus and Christ is well illustrated in the work of Peter Paul Rubens; when we compare his *Prometheus Bound* (fig. 9.3) with his *Deposition of the Cross* from 1612-1614 (fig. 9.11), we see that both works utilise a strong diagonal composition, with the tortured body of the heroic nude as the centre. What Prometheus and Christ also share is the wound in their right side, located between the ribs at the height of the liver that's protected by the ribcage.

Fig. 9.10 Giovanni Antonio Galli (named Spadarino), Christ shows his side wound, 1625-1635, oil paint on canvas, 32,3 × 97,8 cm, The National Gallery, London

The liver is the largest organ in the body and lies against the diaphragm that, like a dome, separates the chest cavity from the abdominal cavity. Directly underneath the right side of this expansion lies the right—and largest—part of the liver, behind the right half of the ribcage. The left part of the liver is smaller and lies further removed from the left rib cage. A wound between the ribs in the right side provides direct access to the liver. For the eagle that tormented Prometheus, this was the perfect location to target the Titan's liver, as is clearly depicted by Rubens in his painting of Prometheus (fig. 9.3). In a large variety of the depictions of the Crucifixion, we see Christ's wound, between the ribs, in his right side as well (fig. 9.12). The blood flowing from the wound suggests that the wound was deep and had injured the liver.

It is remarkable that Rubens, when making an oil paint study for the Deposition, initially placed the wound of Christ on the left side of the body. Somewhere in the process,

Fig. 9.11 *Peter Paul Rubens, Detail of the deposition from the cross. Christ is being carried down from the cross by his followers. On the right side of his ribcage the wound in his side is visible, out of which blood flows down over his torso. 1612-1614, oil paint on canvas, 420 x 320 cm, Onze-Lieve-Vrouwekathedraal, Antwerp*

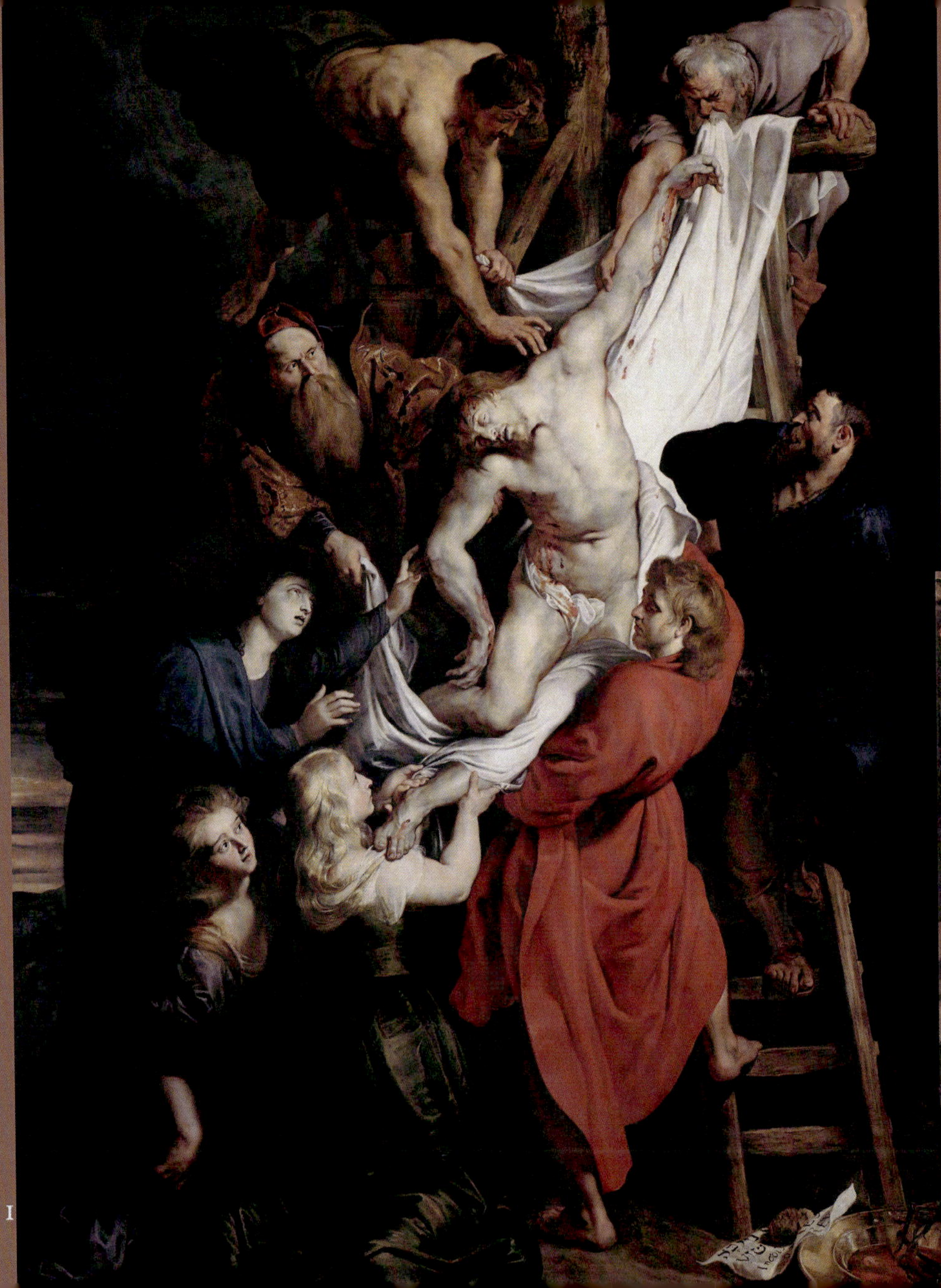

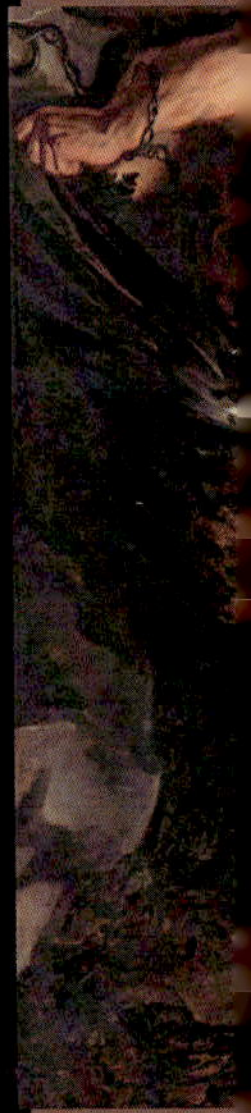

the artist changed his mind and, in the final work, decided to place the wound on the right side, just over the liver. What made Rubens hesitate and change his work? Was Christ stabbed in his liver during his torment, like Prometheus was? Did the liver have symbolic significance in this case?

During his crucifixion, Christ was stabbed in the side with a lance by the Roman centurion Longinus in order to ensure he was truly deceased (John 19:33-37). The evangelist fails to mention in which side of his chest Christ was stabbed. The wound he received from the lance was the fifth, and the last, of the so-called stigmata, and was eventually ascribed important ritual significance. This was in part due to the fact that in the twelfth century, the focus of Christian worship shifted to the humanity of Christ. Saints, like Saint Francis of Assisi, encouraged the worshipers to empathise with Christ's suffering.

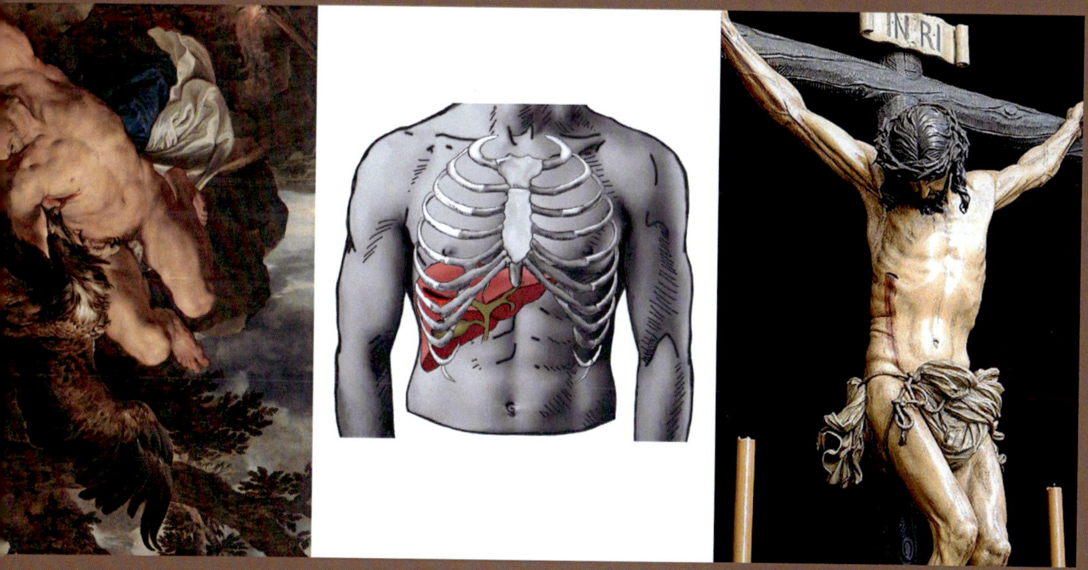

Fig. 9.12 Anatomical relation between the wound on the right side of the ribcage and the liver. From left to right: A reversed image of Prometheus in the painting by Rubens (Fig. 9.3) shows the orientation of the wound in his right side; the anatomical position of the liver directly behind the right half of the ribcage under the diaphragm; the crucified Christ with a bleeding wound in the space between his ribs on the right side of his chest, 1648, Santisimo Cristo de la Buena Muerte, Cádiz

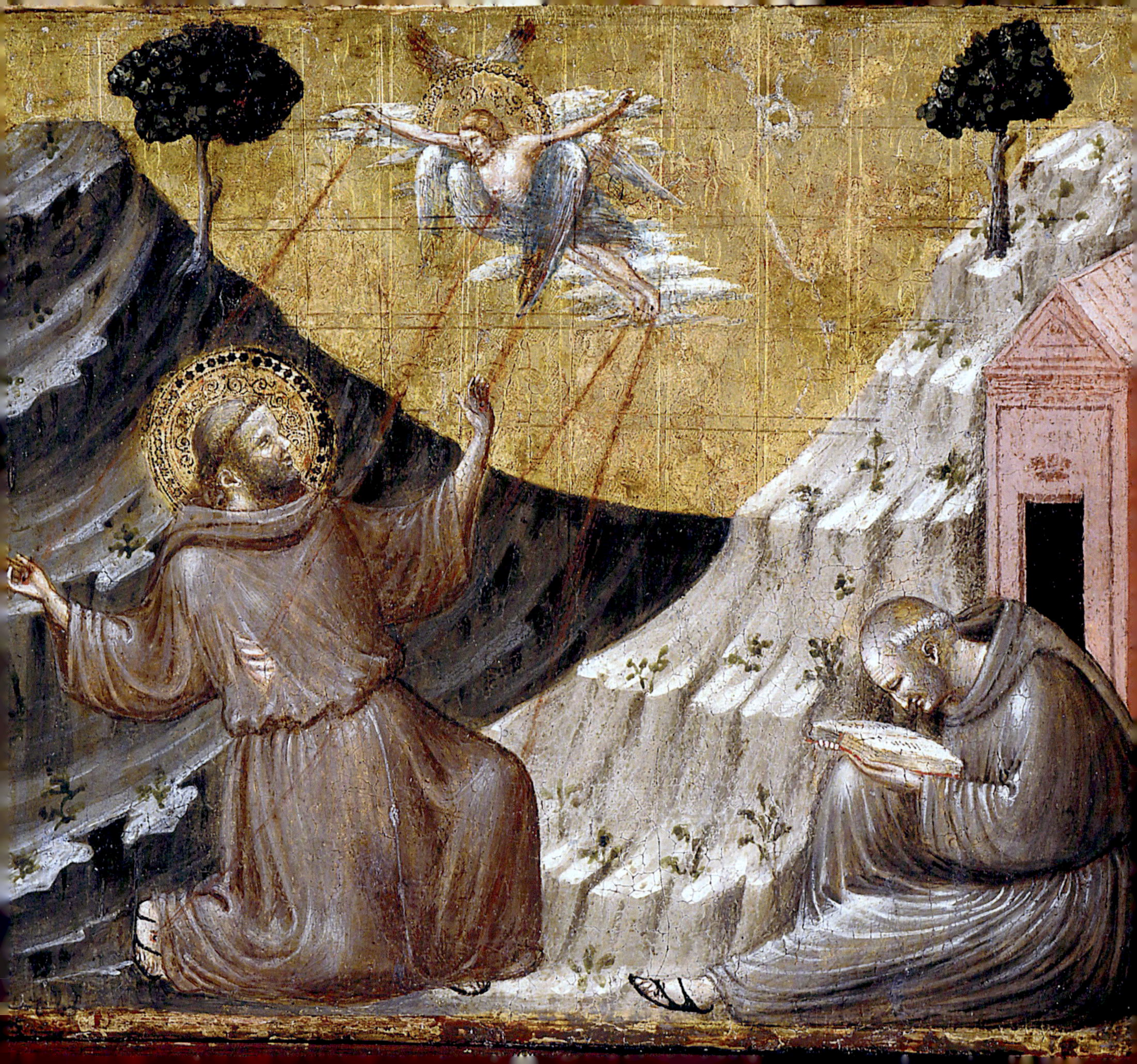

Fig. 9.13 Pietro da Rimini, Saint Francis of Assisi receives the stigmata. A hybrid of a Seraph and Christ appears in the air and beams of light connect the wounds of Christ to the wounds appearing on Saint Francis, among them a beam to the right side of his chest. His habit is torn at that place, showing the wound. C. 1300, Egg tempera on panel, 20,3 × 24,8 cm, Indianapolis Museum of Art, Newfields IN

Francis himself did this to such an extent that he miraculously received the stigmata on his own body (fig. 9.13).

In early depictions of the Crucifixion, the wound was depicted in Christ's left side. This changes in 583 BCE with the *Rabbula Codex* (or the Rabbula Gospels), an illuminated manuscript from Syria. In the illumination in the Codex, the wound was moved to Christ's right side (fig. 9.14). With this illumination, the soldier and his lance, and by extension the wound, became fixed as events occurring on Christ's right side, permanently changing the visual program for this scene. The Syrian monks that produced this manuscript were very influential on the exegesis of the New Testament, and the illuminations they created were rife with symbolism.

There is a threefold explanation of possible factors that may have contributed to the move of the wound from the left to the right side of Christ. The first two explanations are typological in nature: the New Testament was read as the fulfilment of prophecies from the Old Testament, which required certain details to correspond.

One Old Testament prophet, Ezekiel, wrote that he 'saw water flow from the right side of the temple' (Ezk. 47:1-12). The body of Christ was often symbolically read as the temple. This prophecy could only be fulfilled if the wound of Christ was situated at the right side of the body.

The second possible explanation concerns itself explicitly with the liver of Christ. In ancient Judaism, as in other ancient societies, the liver was seen as the seat of life. The Talmud reads: "Man nor beast can survive without liver" (Arakin 20a). It is because of this that the

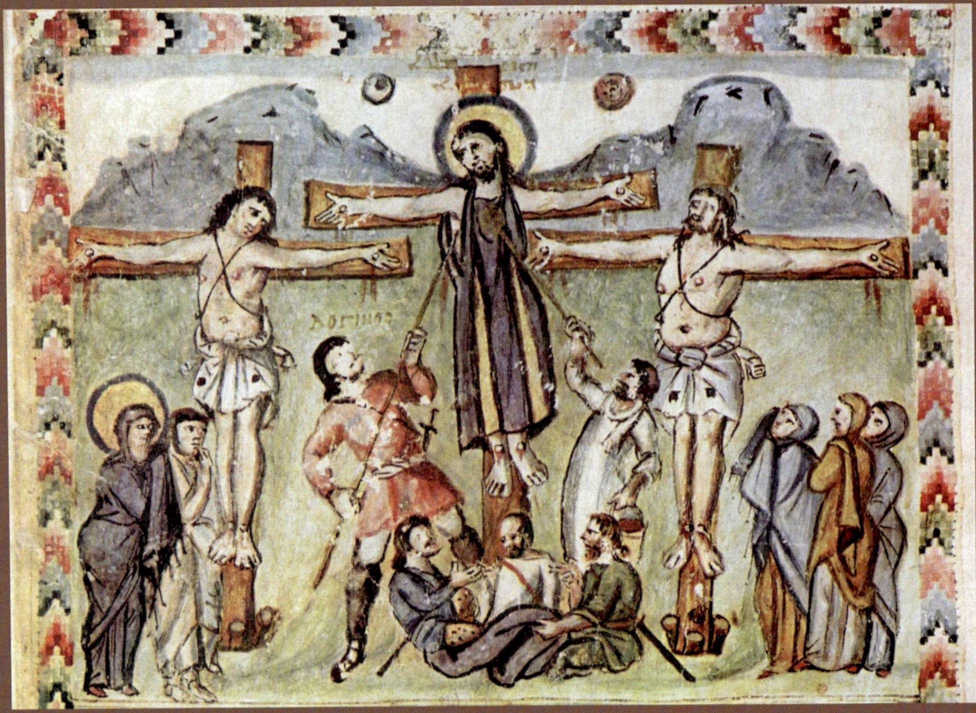

Fig. 9.14 Crucifixion of Christ on mount Calvary. Christ's right side is penetrated with the lance of Longinus, illumination in the Rabbula codex, Beth Zagba (Syria), 586 CE, egg tempera on parchment, 583, 34 x 27 cm, Florence, Biblioteca Medicea-Laurenziana, MS Cod. Pluteus I, 56, fol. 13r

prophet Jeremiah mentions the liver explicitly in his Lamentations: "My eyes are tired of weeping, my intestines are burning, my liver has been spilled over the earth" (lam. 2:11). The Lamentations were originally written to mourn the destruction of Jerusalem in 586 BCE but the later Christian tradition connected this passage of the Old Testament explicitly to the suffering of Christ. Passages from the Lamentations were sung during Lent and on Good Friday, the day that Christ was crucified. The suffering caused by the destruction of Jerusalem was likened to the suffering of Christ. Since the liver is positioned, anatomically speaking, on the right side of the body, and if Christ was hit in his vital organ, his liver, which was then 'spilled out over the earth', the wound had to be situated on his right side so that the prophecy from the Old Testament could be fulfilled as well.

Finally, there's the contributing factor that in Christianity the right side is associated with good and the left side with evil. The blood of Christ, which symbolised salvation, was depicted as flowing from his side wound and because of the qualities associated with good and evil, the blood would have to flow from his right side.

In the later Middle Ages, the wound of Christ acquired its own independent veneration. The blood that flowed from it was said to provide a direct connection between the faithful and Christ because the wine that was drunk at the Eucharist was transubstantiated into the Blood of Christ. In addition to this, the notion developed that the redeeming blood of Christ flowed directly from his heart. This idea was popularised by a group of female saints from the thirteenth and fourteenth centuries, including Saints Gertrude and Mechtilde. The saints describe similar visions where they placed their heads against the chest of Christ and, through the wound in his side, could feel the beating of his heart. It is because of this that, in depictions of the wounds of Christ, the fifth stigma is often depicted as a bleeding heart, and not as

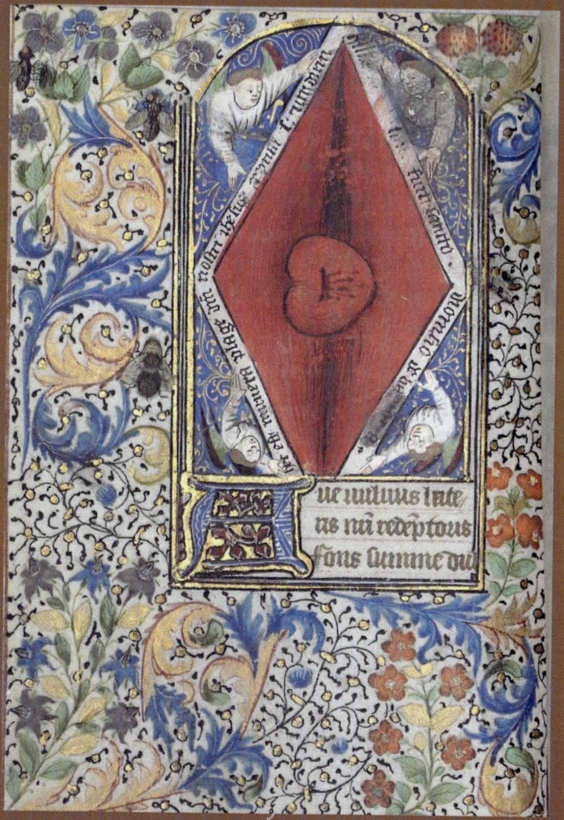

Fig. 9.15 The bleeding heart of Christ. The bleeding heart is depicted in a stylised wound. Illustration from a book of hours Horae ad usum romanum, *15th century, , 125 × 85 mm Bibliothèque nationale de France, Département des manuscrits, Latin 1369, p. 410*

the wound in the right side of the chest. In a fifteenth-century book of hours, we can see the bleeding heart of Christ through the wound (fig. 9.15). Despite the new association between the wound of Christ and the heart of Christ, pictorial tradition mandated that the wound remained on the right side of the body.

This all changed in the seventeenth century, when anatomical knowledge increased and the pictorial arts reflected this anatomical fascination. People became aware that the heart was situated at the left side of the chest. The idea that the wound of Christ was a wound in the heart posed a dilemma to Rubens when painting his *Deposition of the Cross* 1612-14 (fig. 9.11). On one hand, Rubens was dedicated to a scientifically accurate depiction of the human body, in which case a wound in the heart would call for a wound in the left side of the body; on the other hand, the wound of Christ had been depicted on the right side of the body for centuries. Moving the wound to the left side was such a breach of tradition that it was almost seen as heresy. Rubens went back and forth on the two options; in this painting, theological convention won out, but in other paintings he depicted the wound in accordance to the consensus of the position of the heart, on the left side (fig. 9.16).

In a strange coincidence, the centurion Longinus, in punishment for his role in the death of Christ, was locked in a cave. Each night, he was visited by a lion that tore pieces of flesh from his body. But during the day his wounds healed, so that the process could repeat into eternity. The parallel between the punishments of Longinus and Prometheus is quite clear, and leads one to wonder if it was indeed coincidence that both Prometheus and Christ were wounded in their livers.

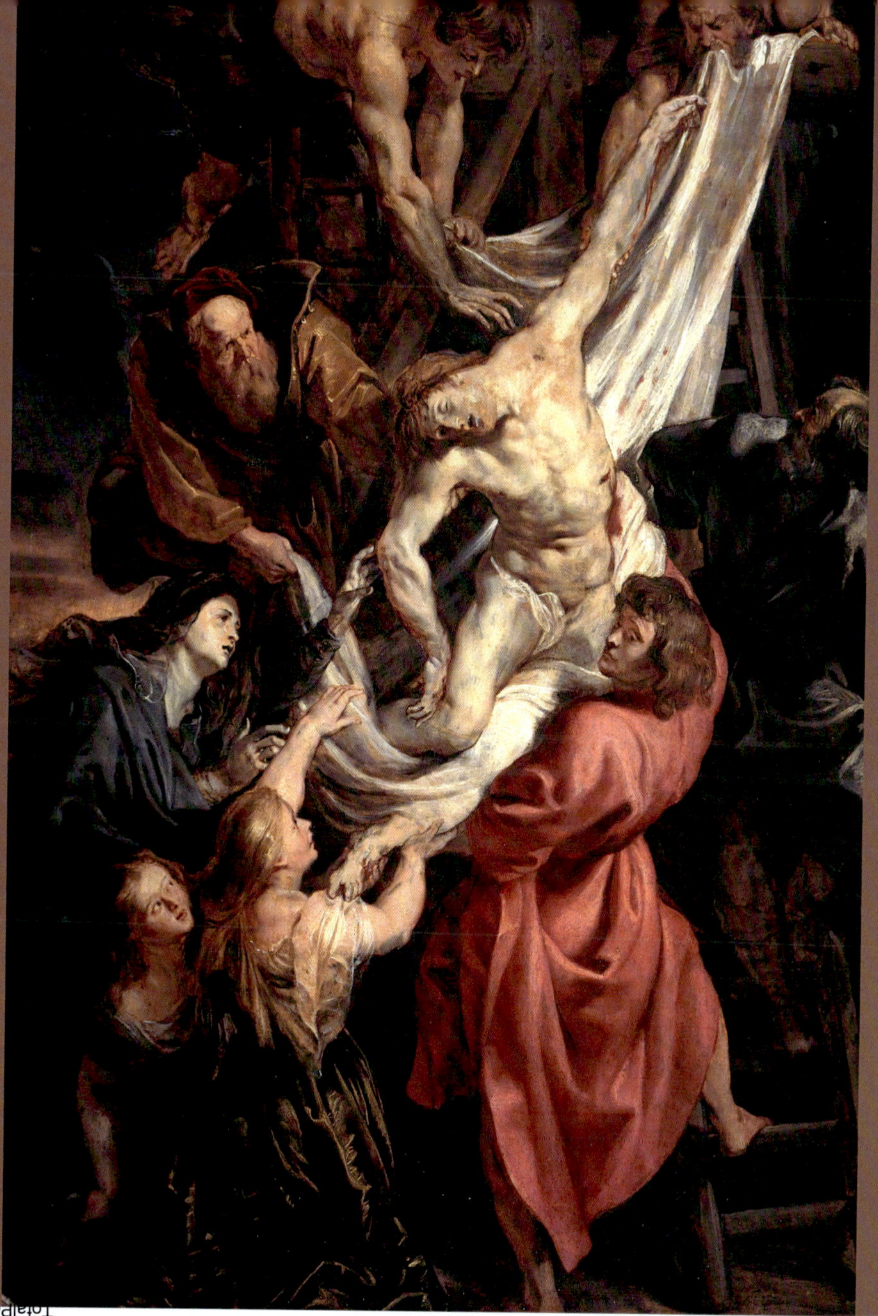

Fig. 9.16 *Peter Paul Rubens, Deposition of the Cross. On this prepatory sketch for the painting from Fig. 9.10, the wound is depicted on the left side of the body. c. 1611-1612, Oil paint on Panel, 115,2 cm x 76,2 cm, Courtauld Institute of Art, London*

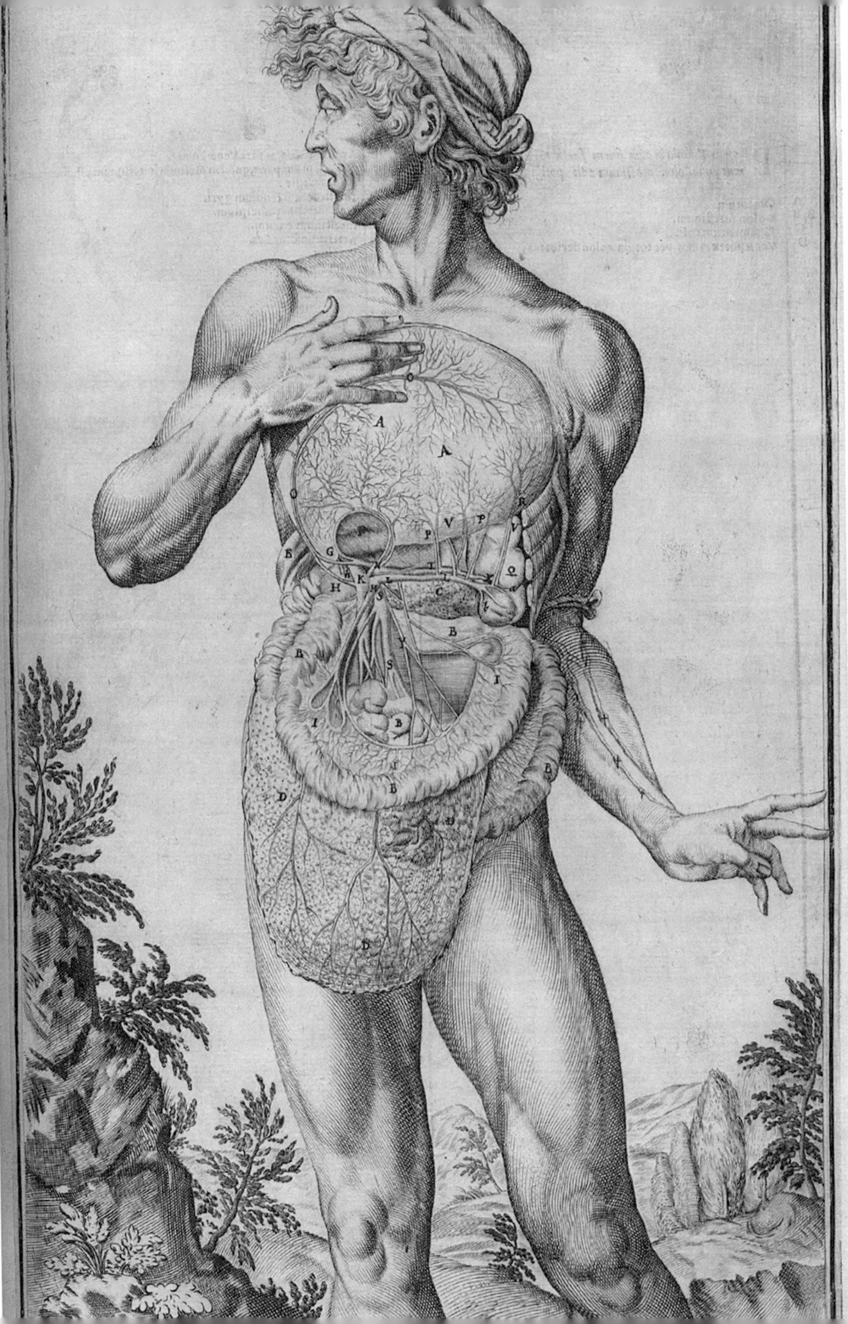

10
THE LIVER IN THE BAROQUE, ACCORDING TO VAN DEN SPIEGEL, GLISSON, AND BIDLOO

Fig 10.0 Man lifts his stomach out of his abdomen revealing the bloodvessels leading to the liver. To the left of the lifted stomach a part of the liver is vissible (E), as well as through a small window in the 'small net' (omentum minus) (P). Figure V-1 from De Humani Corporis Fabrica Libri Decem *by Adriaan van den Spiegel, 1627, Venice*

The quest to find truth through empirical observation that found its origins in the Renaissance came to fruition in the seventeenth century. The publication of the magnum opus of Vesalius, *De Humani Corporis Fabrica*, gave the study of anatomy a scientific basis that was then emulated by many practitioners. The most significant milestone in the beginning of the seventeenth century was the 1628 publication of William Harvey's *De motu cordis et sanguinis in animalibus*, in which this doctor and researcher described the workings of the circulatory system and the heart. Harvey proved that blood was circulated in a closed system in which the valves in the veins ensured that blood would flow in the direction of the heart. This put a definitive end to the tidal theory of Galen, which claimed that blood moved back and forth through veins and then through pores in the cardiac septum, flowing from the right to the left chamber of the heart. Although Harvey experienced some initial pushback from a handful of traditional Galenists, who called him a quack, his theory would soon be embraced and confirmed by many others.

Simultaneously, attention shifted from morphology to the functional aspects of anatomical research in the seventeenth century. There was a desire, among those who propagated a more modern science, to understand the function of organs and anatomical structures. This can be seen in art, as in the famous painting by Rembrandt, *The Anatomy Lesson of Dr. Nicolaes Tulp* (1632). In the work, Dr. Tulp demonstrates the musculature of the arm, using forceps to stretch the tendons in the opened arm, his left hand pulling the tendon to cause movement in the thumb and index finger of the body of convicted felon Aris Kindt.

In the seventeenth century, several important anatomical treatises were published that cast new light on the liver. In the books by Adriaan Van den Spiegel (1627), Francis Glisson (1654) and Govert Bidloo (1685), we see how knowledge about the anatomy of the liver developed further, moving from a rudimentary idea of the appearance of the liver to a true to nature depiction of both the external shape as well as the internal structures of the organ.

THE ANATOMICAL ATLAS OF ADRIAAN VAN DEN SPIEGEL

Adriaan van den Spiegel (1578-1625), also known as 'Spigelius' in Latin, was born in Brussels to an army surgeon (fig. 10.1). He studied medicine in Louvain and Leiden, studying under, among others Petrus Pauw (1564-1617), professor in anatomy and botany at Leiden University. Inspired by Pauw, Van den Spiegel showed a special interest in dissection early on in his study and career. In 1601, Van den Spiegel applied to the famous University of Padua, where he advanced his studies as a doctor and an anatomist. In 1616, he was appointed professor of dissection and surgery at Padua and taught at the famed *Theatrum Anatomicum* of the medical faculty.

In Padua, van den Spiegel worked on an anatomical atlas for an extensive period, which he titled *De Humani Corporis Fabrica Libri Decem*, emulating the famous atlas by Andreas Vesalius (see chapter eight). By doing so, he wanted to compare himself to his famous predecessor and fellow countryman, who preceded him as the chair of anatomy at Padua. Van den Spiegels' anatomical atlas, con-

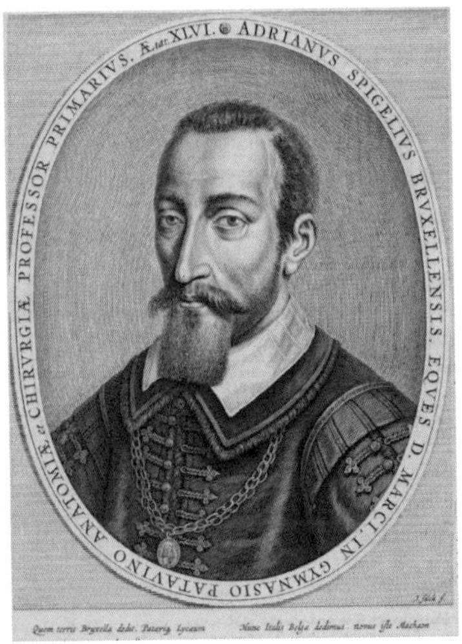
ADRIANVS SPIGELIVS BRVXELLENSIS. EQVES D. MARCI. IN GYMNASIO PATAVINO ANATOMIÆ et CHIRVRGIÆ PROFESSOR PRIMARIVS. Ætat. XLVI.

Fig. 10.1 Adriaan van den Spiegel (1578-1625). Portrait from Opera Omnia, *A. Spiegelius, published by J. Blaeu, 1645, Amsterdam, copper engraving by Jeremias Falck.*

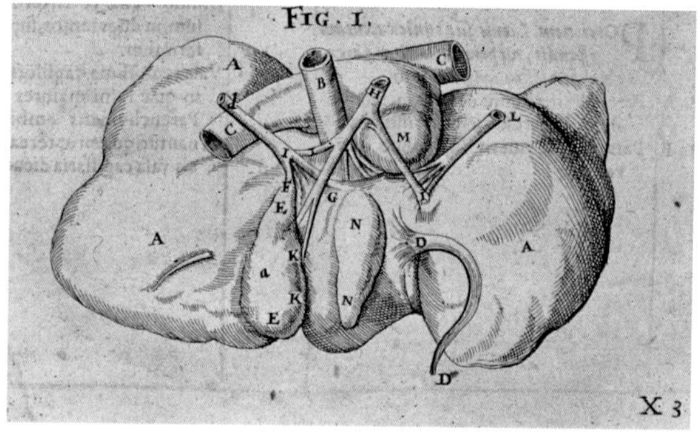

Fig. 10.2 Illustration of the liver from the Fabrica *by Adriaan van den Spiegel. The lower side of the liver is shown in a reversed position, with the round side of the gallbladder (E) turned downwards. This image is the first to depict the small liver lobe at the backside of the liver, the lobus caudatus (M), now also known as the lobus Spigelii*

sisting of ten parts, was published in 1627 – two years after his death – and was richly decorated with illustrated plates that were partially taken from the *Tabulae Anatomicae* (Venice, 1627) of the anatomist Giulio Cesare Casseri (1552-1616) – his immediate predecessor in Padua. In this book, Van den Spiegel was the first to describe the *lobus caudatus*, a small lobe at the back of the liver, that had played such an important role for the Etruscan seers when they studied their sheeps' livers to read the future (see chapter four). This lobe obtained its name—and continues to be known—under the eponym 'lobus Spigelli' (even though the lobe was already depicted on the same plate in the earlier book by Casseri) (fig. 10.2). Van den Spiegel died in 1625 from an infected wound and, as was shown by a dissection of his own body, from an abscess underneath the *lobus caudatus,* the lobe that would later bear his name (*lobus Spigelli*).

THE 'ANATOMIA HEPATIS' BY FRANCIS GLISSON

The first monograph on the anatomy and function of the liver is the book *Anatomia Hepatis*, written by the Englishman Francis Glisson (1598-1677) and published in 1654 in Amsterdam. Francis Glisson was born in Bristol and studied to become a doctor at Caius College, Cambridge (fig. 10.3). He became

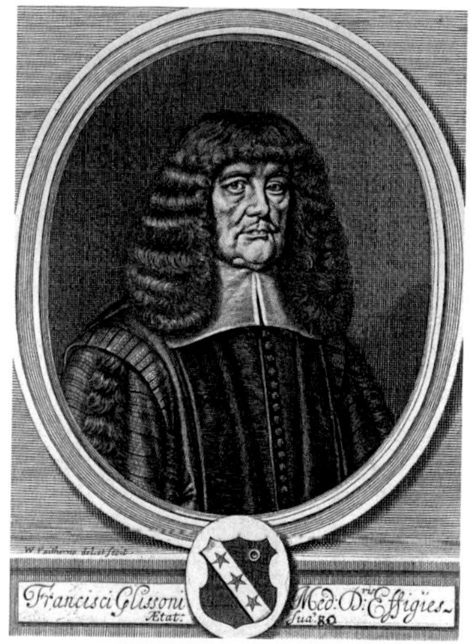

Fig. 10.3 Francis Glisson (1598-1677), title page from Tractatus de ventriculo et intestinis, *F. Glisson, 1677, London, copper engraving by W. Faithorne*

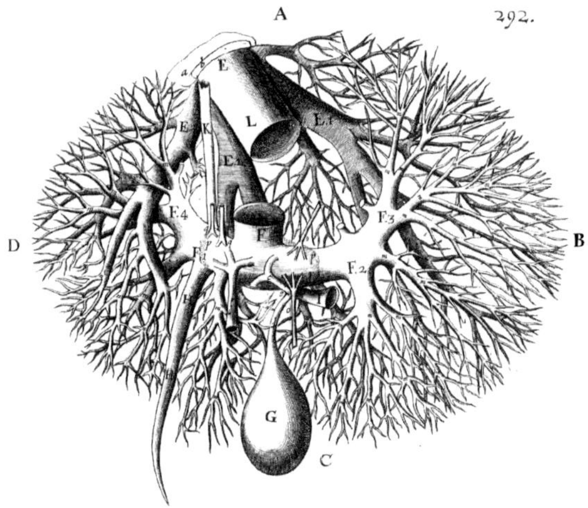

Fig. 10.4 During his research Glisson utilised the injection method where the blood vessels were injected with milk and the surrounding liver tissue was removed. With this 'excarnation technique' he was able to create a three-dimensional cast of the blood vessel system and bile ducts in the liver. The liver is depicted reversed in this image with the round side of the gallbladder (G) directed downward, as was the case in the illustration by Van der Spiegel (Fig. 10.2)

professor of medicine at Cambridge, where he dedicated himself to anatomy, physiology and philosophy. As a contemporary of William Harvey (1578-1657), who, as previously mentioned, discovered the circulatory system, Glisson examined the veins in the liver by injecting them with water or milk and then removing the liver tissue, thus creating a cast of the network of veins (fig. 10.4). By doing so, he managed to demonstrate that there was a connection between the portal venous system and the lower *vena cava*.

Using the same method, Glisson documented the network of the bile ducts including the gallbladder and the excretory bile duct to the duodenum, the part of the gut following the stomach. A purifying property was appointed to bile. In addition to this designation, bile was thought to produce warmth. Glisson also described the phenomenon where gallstones can become lodged in the bile ducts and cause severe pain. His name, however, was appointed to the so-called 'fibrous capsule of Glisson,' a thin layer of fibrous tissue that surrounds the liver and extends to the internal structure of the organ where it encapsulates the bundles of veins and bile ducts.

THE ANATOMIA HUMANI CORPORIS BY GOVERT BIDLOO

Govert Bidloo (1649-1717) was born in Amsterdam, the son of an apothecary (fig. 10.5). He trained to become a surgeon under, among others, the famous Frederik Ruysch, who was appointed teacher (*praelector anatomiae*) by the guild of surgeons in order to educate the apprentices in surgery in the anatomical sciences. In 1682, Bidloo obtained the title of doctor at the University of Franeker. He wasn't solely known as surgeon and anatomist but also – and perhaps primarily – as a successful playwright and poet. Bidloo assembled an anatomical atlas consisting of one hundred fifty high quality engravings by the esteemed artist Gerard de Lairesse (1640-1711), producing the work, *Anatomia Humani Corporis* (1685). The amount of detail in the illustrations is what truly sets this atlas apart from others of its kind. The texts, however, are relatively spare – a reason why the atlas was lauded more for its artistic value than its scientific impact.

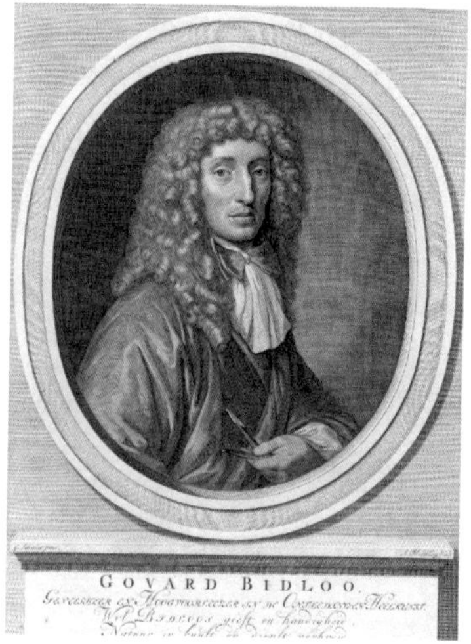

Fig. 10.5 Govert Bidloo (1649-1713), copper engraving, The National Gallery, London

Bidloo's passion for theatre and dramatics is reflected in the unfettered composition of the anatomic plates, where the parts of the body that are being dissected are covered with pieces of cloth and the preparations are displayed in the same way they would be on the dissection table, including all the pins, hooks, and needles. This was a decisive move from traditional depictions of cadavers and anatomical preparation, which showed the scene in an idealised form without any of the mutilations inflicted upon the body by the process of dissection.

An astounding case of plagiarism occurred in 1698 when the English surgeon and anatomist William Cowper (1666-1709) published his own edition of the atlas in which he shamelessly included the same series of plates by Gerard de Lairesse without even mentioning Bidloo's name. Even the title page remained the same, simply replacing Bidloo's name in the author's medallion with Cowper's. A fiery dispute ensued that would drag on for years and end without any satisfactory conclusion for Bidloo. One argument that can be made for Cowper's copy is that the accompanying texts that he added were of a far higher quality, which made the atlas a more applicable and indeed useful tool. Bidloo's future didn't suffer for Cowper's act, as he became the personal physician of Stadtholder, and eventual King of England, William III (1650-1702), also widely known as William of Orange.

In his anatomical atlas, Bidloo depicts the liver—with part of the diaphragm still attached to it—as it appears outside of the body and on display (fig. 10.6). Wooden pins in the *vena cava* and in the portal vein signify the position and direction of these important structures. In the image, the liver is reversed: the lower side shows the gallbladder pointing downwards, which reminds us of the Etruscan model many centuries earlier (see chapter three, fig. 3.2 (give the figure number for the image of the liver in the Etruscan context). From an anatomical viewpoint, the right and left liver lobes are reversed as well. This total reversal is the result of the reproduction of the original drawing by de Lairesse as an engraving. The mechanical reproduction process will result in a mirrored image if the original wasn't mirrored when being engraved in the copper plate. In the case of this liver, the image wasn't properly inverted during the production process and then directly copied onto the copper plate, resulting in a mirrored image of the liver. This technical mistake occurred more often in this printing technique, but was less noticeable in symmetrical organs.

In the Baroque, the urge for scientific depth that had arisen in the Renaissance, further matured and produced some fine anatomical atlases. As much detailed these were, the anatomical depictions and annotations of the liver were largely descriptive, lacking understanding of it's function. In the following century, the functional features of the liver were explored, ushering scientists into a new era of medical research.

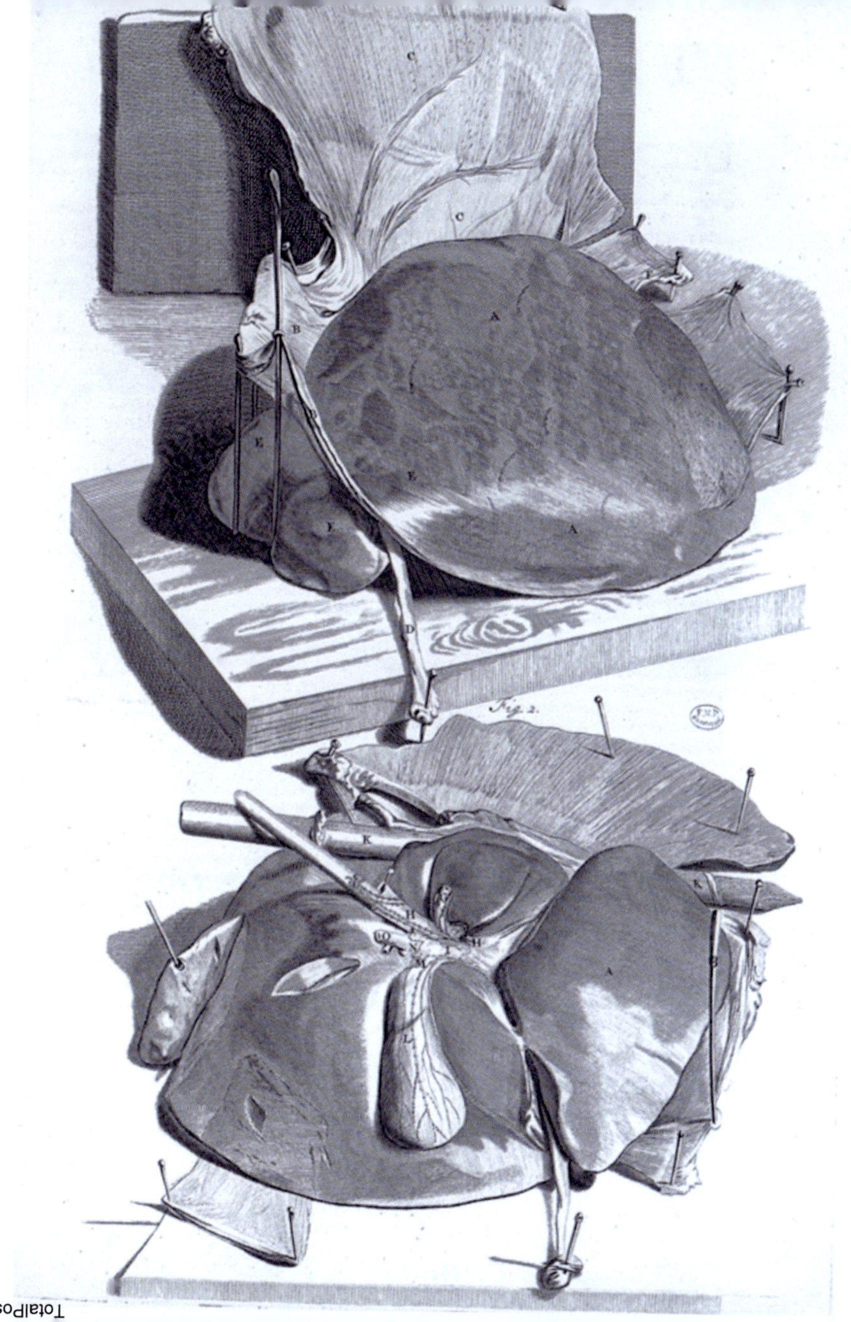

Fig. 10.6 The liver as depicted in Anatomia Humani Corporis, *the anatomical atlas by Govert Bidloo and illustrated by Gerard de Lairesse. This liver is depicted reversed, with the gallbladder pointing downwards, as well as mirrored due to a mistake in the reproduction process from drawing to engraving, causing the anatomical left and right liver lobe to be reversed.*

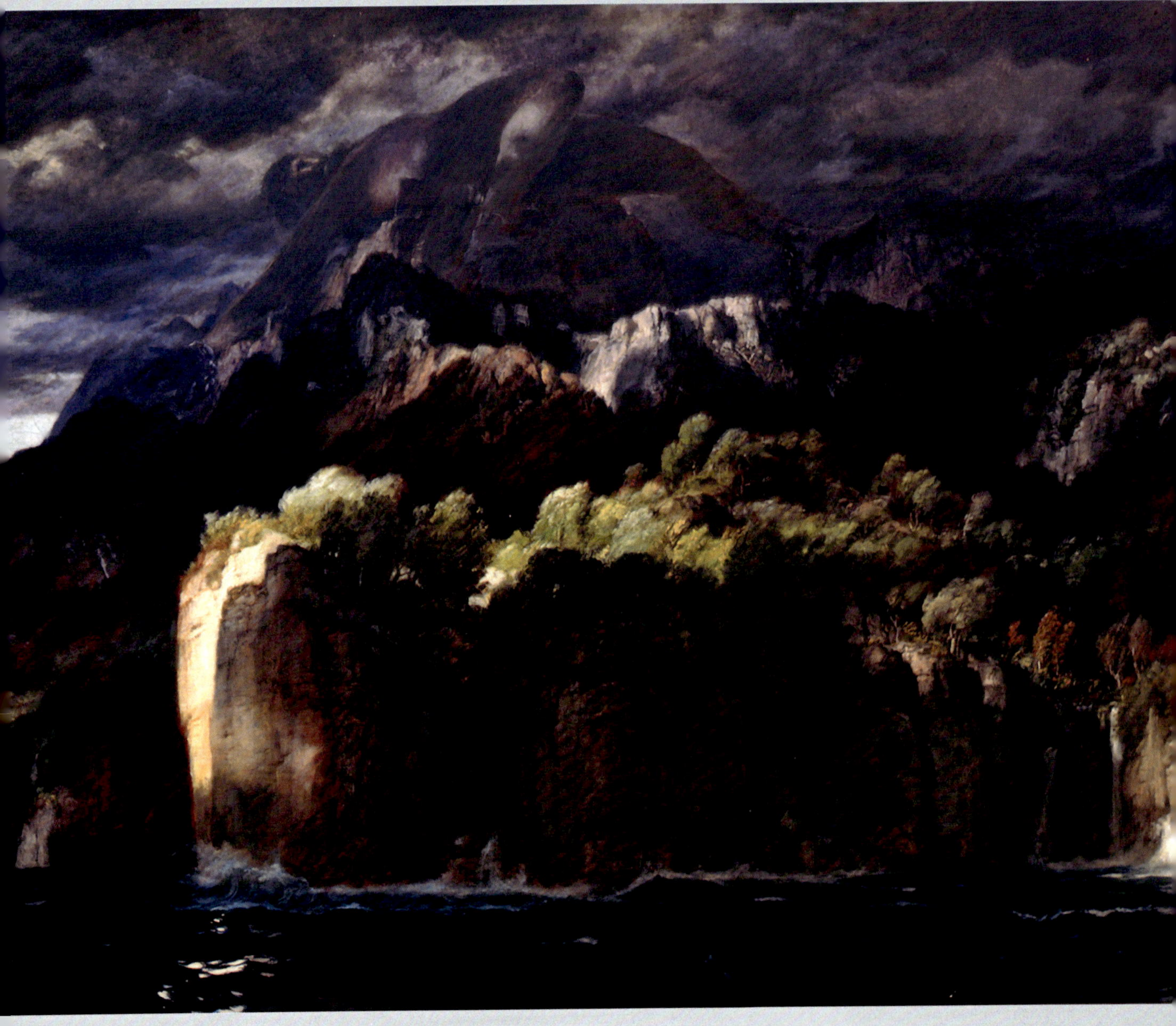

11
PROMETHEUS AND MODERNITY

In the previous chapters, the art historical stylistic periodisation encompasses quite large stretches of time. Despite undeniable technical progress within artistic practice, the circumstances of patronage and the climate around art commission and production remained relatively uniform. Nobility, monarchy, and the Church remained present within society and continued to represent the most significant client base for prominent artists. By the end of the eighteenth century, this 'client base' started to change. A succession of political, scientific, and industrial revolutions heralded the dawn of a new era. While preceding centuries are generally referred to as 'pre-modern' or 'early-modern', these developments characterise the advent of what is now called 'modernity'.

The initial interest in Prometheus in the modern period was philosophical and literary in nature. Countless figures of political philosophy used Prometheus as an aspirational or allegorical figure. Thomas Hobbes (1588-1679), a defender of absolutism, cast a negative judgement on Prometheus. Hobbes saw in the Titan the rebel who challenged absolute power, punished for his crime against the philosopher's idea of a natural order that gave all power to the monarch. On the other hand, the Enlightenment thinker and poet Voltaire (1694-1778), a prominent figure during the French Revolution, saw Prometheus as

Fig. 11.0 Arnold Böcklin, Prometheus landscape. High in a mountainous landscape almost entirely hidden by storm clouds, a giant Prometheus is chained to a mountain. 1883, oil paint on canvas, 150 x 116 cm, private collection

an aspirational figure who, like a revolutionary rebel, had bravely stood up to Zeus and against tyrannical despotism.

In the realm of literature, there was a great interest in Prometheus as well. Johann Wolfgang von Goethe (1749-1832) wrote a poetic ode dedicated to the Titan and a play (unfinished). Goethe recognised himself and his literary process in Prometheus who, isolated from the gods, created humankind in his workplace. This was in line with a new-found idolisation of artistic genius that characterised the artistic climate, in the broadest sense, of Goethe's time. Philosophers, artists, writers, and musicians alike fostered this image of gifted creative spirits, isolated exactly because of their genius. Goethe was one of the first to turn to the myth of Prometheus in this matter, but he would not be alone.

Without prior knowledge of the work of Goethe, three English writers came to the Prometheus subject—these writers were part of a literary friend group consisting of Lord Byron (1788-1824), Percy Byshe Shelley (1792-1822) and his wife Mary Shelley (1797-1851) were all fascinated by Prometheus. The Titan is a recurring figure in Byron's poems and Percy Shelley wrote a complete lyrical drama on the Titan, following in the footsteps of Aeschylus. Shelley made the Aeschylus narrative his own; he wanted to explore what might be contained in the parts of the tragedy that had been lost, not with the intention of reproducing a faithful reconstruction of the tragedy, but rather emulating it according to his own artistic vision. To Shelley, Prometheus was the champion of mankind and he could not accept any reconciliation between Prometheus and Zeus, the oppressor of mankind – a plot point that was likely included in the resolution of Aeschylus' play. Shelley elevated Prometheus to the status of 'Romantic hero,' an ideal that artists should mirror themselves after. This mirroring was something that these Byron and Shelley embodied and encouraged to an even greater extent than Goethe. It was not only in his status as 'isolated genius' that Prometheus became the mirror of the artist; the Titan's rebellion against established order and willingness to suffer on behalf of his creation—and that creation and suffering were thus intrinsically linked—were all ideals of the nineteenth-century artist.

Unlike her male compatriots, Mary Shelley took a different approach. Rather than cast the Titan as a Romantic hero, she transformed Prometheus into Victor Frankenstein, the main character in her 1818 book *Frankenstein; or, The Modern Prometheus*. Here, Prometheus doesn't exactly appear to be a hero. A more extensive look at of Mary Shelley's subversion of the theme of Prometheus as a Romantic hero follows in the insert accompanying this chapter.

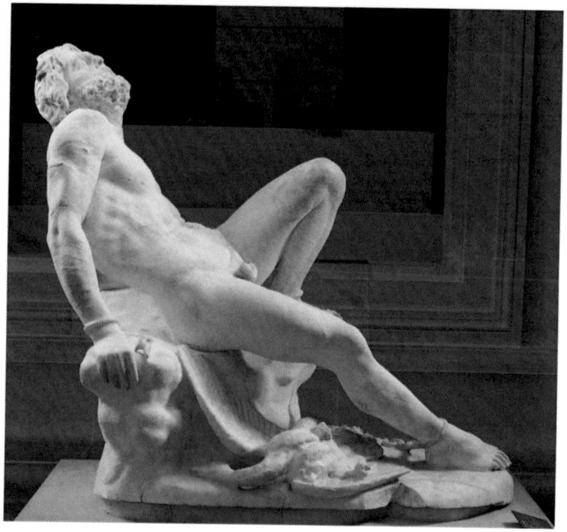

Fig. 11.1 Jean Jacques Pradier, Prometheus bound. The eagle has been slain and lies at Prometheus' feet. 1827, marble, 152 x 170 x 80 cm, Louvre, Paris

PROMETHEUS AS THE EMBODIMENT OF THE ENLIGHTENMENT

Where the visual arts are concerned, it took slightly longer for Prometheus to become an archetypical Romantic hero. In the early decades of the nineteenth century, the art world was governed by the strong normative standards of so-called 'academic art.' These standards were developed by the *Académie des Beaux-Arts in Paris*, an institution that initially served the French court and, after the Revolution, was adopted by the state. The artists that received their education at the *Académie* were trained to uphold *Académie* standards until they were deemed ready to make their debut in the famous 'salons,' where their work was exhibited alongside that of established artists, and further scrutinised by both judges from the *Académie* and the general public.

The style associated with the *Académie* is generally conservative and traditional—as a reaction on the exuberance of the art of the Baroque, the *Académie* preferred the more sober Neoclassicism. While preserving the lessons on anatomy and dramatic lighting that were gleaned from the Baroque, Neoclassical art set out to introduce more serenity and balance into its compositions, emulating the Renaissance return to the classical. The preferred antique source shifted once again from Hellenistic back to classical art.

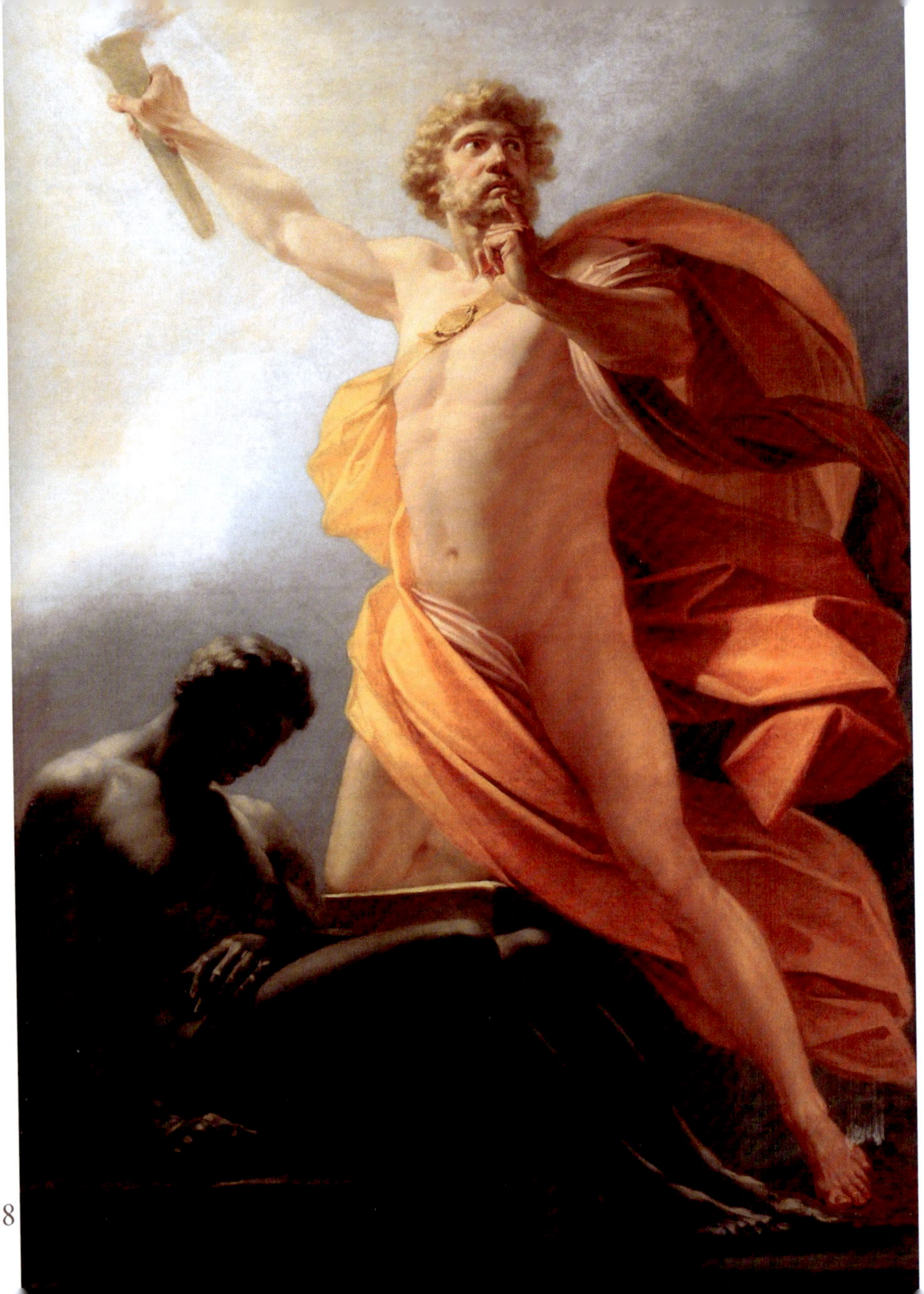

Fig. 11.2 Heinrich Füger, Prometheus brings the fire to mankind. Humanity is represented as a clay statue in the shadowy foreground, still to be animated with the fire. 1817, oil paint on canvas, 221 x 156 cm, Liechtenstein Museum, Vienna

A

prime example of a Neoclassical depiction of Prometheus can be found in the statue that sculptor Jean-Jacques Pradier (1790-1852) made of the Titan in 1827 (fig. 11.1). The work was displayed in the Tuileries Garden in Paris, but has since been moved to the Louvre to protect it from erosion and deterioration. Pradier deemed Prometheus a fitting subject for a 'history piece.' History painting was the highest form of art according to the hierarchy of genres utilised in academic painting, surpassing genre pieces, landscapes, still lifes and portraits. Pradier transposed this hierarchy, applying its dictation of painting styles to sculpture. Pradier – following in the footsteps of Rubens and Titian – depicted Prometheus naturalistically and—as was established during the Baroque—at the moment of the Titan's greatest torture, chained to the Caucasus, leaning backwards and with one knee pulled up. There are, however, marked differences between this neoclassical statue and the Baroque works of the preceding century, where all limbs seem to be contorted in pain, and Prometheus often appears to scream. In Pradier's statue, Prometheus turns his gaze to the sky – looking to Zeus – but his suffering face shows no rage against his captor; his entire demeanour is calm and dignified as he undergoes his punishment, a Neoclassical answer of patient endurance to the drama of the baroque.

Although the famous *Académie des Beaux-Arts* was situated in Paris, this academic style wasn't solely a French phenomenon. Many European countries were home to similar institutes that propagated like-minded styles. Take for example the Austrian *Akademie der bildenden Künste Wien*, where the painter Heinrich Füger was professor and vice-director. Füger was a neoclassicist *pur sang*, which is shown in his monumental painting of Prometheus in the act of bringing fire to mankind (fig. 11.2). The image reflects the ideas of philosophers who saw Prometheus as an aspirational figure and made him the embodiment of reason, rationality and the ideals of progress associated with the Enlightenment. Prometheus is depicted in a triumphant return from Olympus, bringing the stolen fire to the slumped-over human, who is still enveloped in shadows; the Titan is literally enlightening the human. The male figure representing humanity is depicted in monochrome, which, when paired with his soft and limp posture, gives the suggestion that this is lifeless clay. Prometheus holds his finger to his chin. What is the meaning of his gesture? Is he in deep contemplation, is he calling the attention of the? spectator to his monumental action or is he hushing us to remind us of the covert nature of his action? If it is a whisper, it forms a stark contrast to the rest of his posture: the Titan's bold strides can hardly be called stealthy.

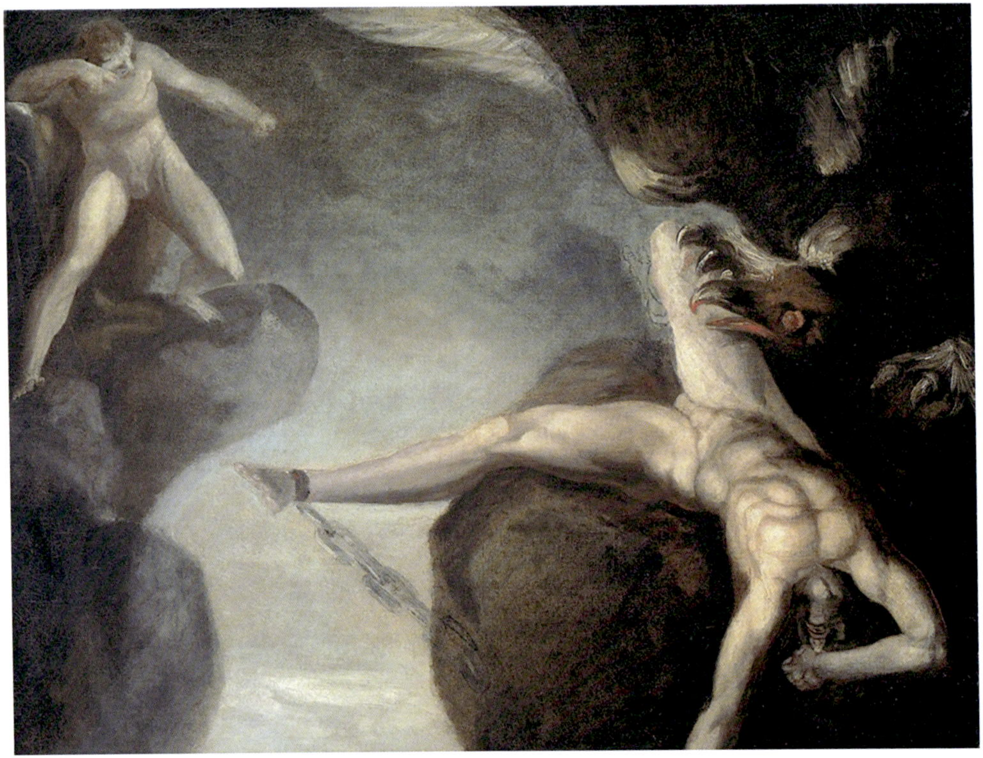

Fig. 11.3 Henry Fuseli, Prometheus is rescued by Herakles. In the upper-left Herakles aims a – yet to be painted – bow at the monstrous eagle that is bending over Prometheus. C. 1781-1785, oil paint on canvas, 63 x 75 cm, sold in auction at Christie's, London, 14 April 1992, nr. LOT 27 SALE 4739

MODERNITY AND ITS DISCONTENTS: ROMANTIC ESCAPISM

Not everyone was so eager to embrace the rapid societal developments of the nineteenth century. At the outset of the nineteenth century, the negative consequences of the burgeoning Industrial Revolution that continued from the previous century started to become apparent: poverty, extensive pollution in rapidly industrialising and expanding cities and urbanisation all contributed to growing malcontent. There was a demand for alternatives to the ideals of the Enlightenment and this need was met by what is now called 'romanticism.' Romantic works are characterised by a strong emphasis on individual creativity and emotion.

In England, where the Industrial Revolution took place slightly earlier than in the rest of Europe, we have already discussed how writers made Prometheus into a 'romantic hero', a symbol of this movement. The Romantic Movement extended to the visual arts. Here, it formed as a reaction to the strict and formalistic academic art, which aimed to embody the ideals of the Enlightenment, but was deemed restrictive and dogmatic by the Romantics. Romantic art tends to be characterised by various types of escapism. Artists turned away from their lived realities and instead found solace in an escapism that can be roughly divided into five categories: the grandeur of nature, the distant past, far-off places, the magical and the mystical and the subconscious. Because emphasis was placed on individualism, romanticism was an attitude rather than a distinct style. Within the Romantic Movement many artists displayed a fascination for the notion of the 'sublime,' the aesthetic theory that we discussed in the chapter on the baroque. Instead of focussing on harmonic beauty, as was the case with neoclassicism, there was room to experiment with the expressive properties of the dark and macabre.

One of the pioneers of the Romantic Movement was the Swiss-British artist Henry Fuseli (1741-1825). His 1781-85 oil painting *Prometheus Freed by Hercules*, (Herakles) clearly demonstrates the contrast between the Romantic Movement and the established neoclassical art of the *Académie* (fig. 11.3). Prometheus is sprawled in a painful and unnatural pose over the rocks. In the upper-left corner, Herakles approaches; the hero is posed

Fig. 11.4 Design by Theodore von Holst, engraving by William Chevalier, frontispiece for Mary Shelley's Frankenstein, (third edition, 1831). Victor Frankenstein flees his room, abhorred by his creation. The newly awakened creature lies on the floor in a dazed state, surrounded by scientific instruments and paraphernalia that got knocked over. British Library, London, MS: 1135.a.9.(1.)

MARY SHELLEY'S *FRANKENSTEIN; OR, THE MODERN PROMETHEUS*

In the romantic period, Prometheus was elevated to the status of a 'romantic hero.' Artists and writers alike projected themselves onto the plight of the Titan, who suffered nobly for the humans he created. Interestingly, we see a nearly opposite approach in one of the most famous gothic novels ever written, often praised as the birth of the science fiction genre: *Frankenstein* by Mary Shelley. She gave her novel, published in 1818, the alternative title *The Modern Prometheus* and cast the Titan as a prototypical anti-hero.

The role of Prometheus in the novel was located in the main character, Victor Frankenstein. Victor, an ambitious doctoral student in the natural sciences department of the University of Ingolstadt, has the ambition to restore life to an artificially created body composed of various parts of different corpses. Mary Shelley's narrative sets out to demonstrate that the act of creation, in any shape or form, also mandates a responsibility for that which has been created. Victor's experiment was successful, but the features of his creature seemed so uncanny and unnatural when animated that they filled him with horror, and, instead of taking responsibility for what he created, he fled and abandoned the creature in his lab. The creature fled in turn, orphaned and lost, into the unknown and hostile world. Here, the paths of Frankenstein and Prometheus seem to diverge. Prometheus took responsibility for the humans he created; by bringing them fire, he simultaneously enlightened and 'educated' mankind. Mary Shelley's Victor-Prometheus is only half Prometheus: he wanted to create at all costs, but did not take the responsibility to take care for his creation's education.

During his search for his creator, the creature was ostracised and cast out at every turn, growing from an innocent blank slate into an embittered and resentful being. Finally, he turns to violence himself, his first victim being Victor Frankenstein's youngest brother, after which he dedicates his life to tormenting his creator until the Victor acknowledges him and his loneliness and makes him a bride. The creature's incessant cruelty is comparable with the eagle that visits Prometheus again and again. The slow murder of all of Victor's loved ones is like a metaphorical tearing out of his heart or liver. Finally, this cruelty finds its apex in the murder of Victor's bride, Elizabeth, on their wedding night.

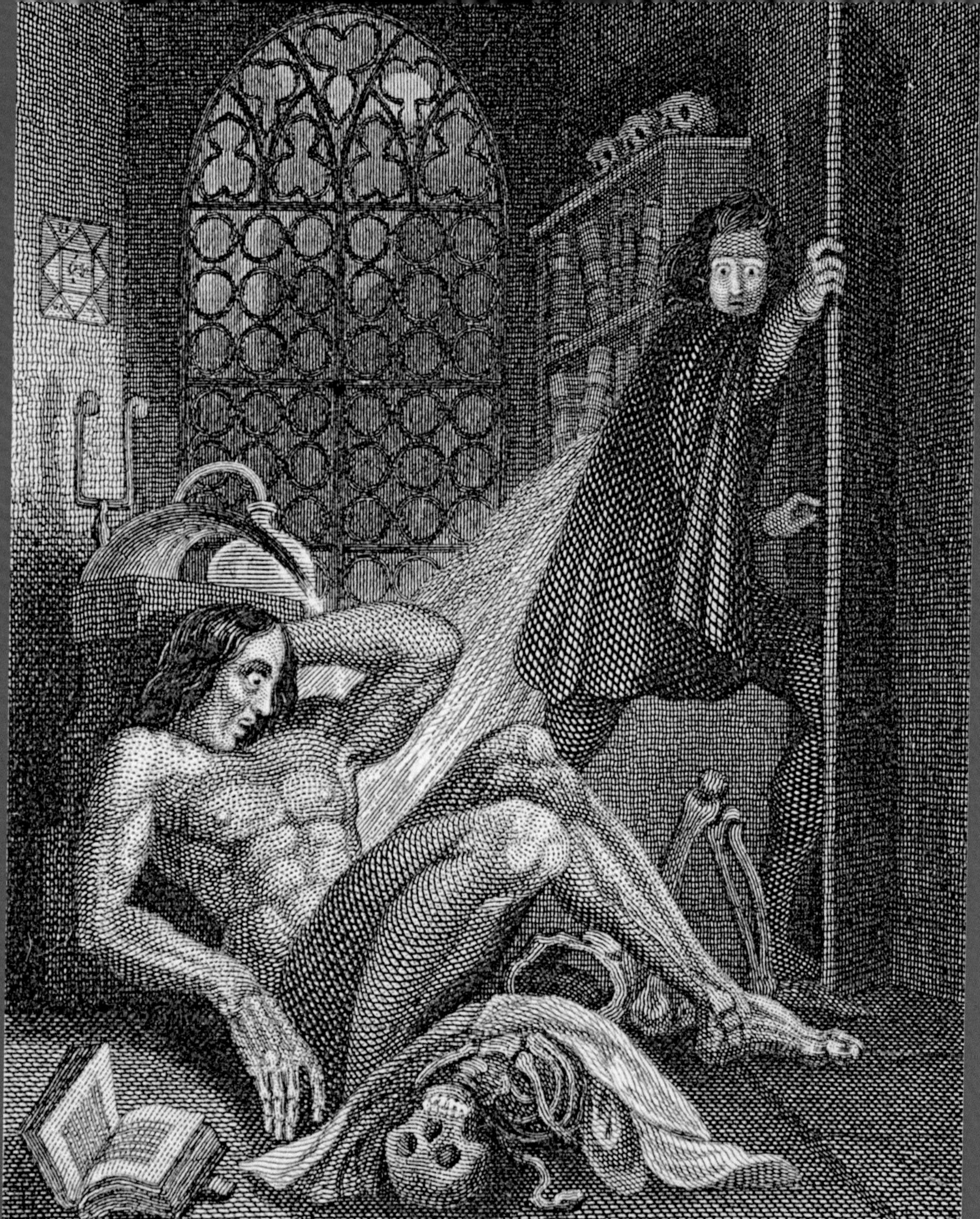

Victor turns from passive endurance of his creature's actions to active pursuit of his creation. The mad hunt ends on the wide plane of a frozen sea of ice in the far north. Victor is rescued by the young Captain Walton, to whom he tells his story before succumbing to his exhaustion. Before his death, Frankenstein begs Walton to kill the creature should he come across it. Despite the wishes of his dying friend, Walton does not follow the request. When he finds the creature on his ship, weeping over Victor's dead body, Walton understands what Victor himself never did: that the fate of creature and creator are closely intertwined and that the creature's malice does not exist outside of his creator.

In fact, the creature himself declares that now that Frankenstein's fate has been fulfilled, his own life will come to an end as well. The creature disappears back onto the sea of ice with the solemn resolution to end his own life. Creator and creation were not opposites in this story, but rather mirror images that reflected each other. Frankenstein was a modern Prometheus, but his creation was as much a suffering hero as he was.

The engraving that adorns the frontispiece of Mary Shelley's book shows the creature naked in the foreground, surrounded by toppled scientific instruments and all sorts of paraphernalia. With large and wild eyes, the freshly animated creature slowly gains awareness of the world surrounding him. The young Victor Frankenstein flees through a back door, abhorring his creation. The creature is depicted as a large heroic nude, in the same pose with one knee bent and one leg outstretched that we have seen in depictions of the heroic and suffering Prometheus. The depiction, dominated by the large heroic nude, is redolent of Jacob Jordaens' 1640 painting *Prometheus Bound* discussed in chapter nine (fig. 9.7). In Jordaens' work, Prometheus is the heroic nude at the forefront, while Hermes makes his exit in the background. On the illustration of *Frankenstein*, however, these roles seem to be reversed: the creature takes the position of the suffering hero, while Frankenstein, despite the fact that he fulfills the role of Prometheus in the novel, is in the position of Hermes, quickly fleeing the scene. In this way, the illustration mirrors the subtle message of the book: creator and creation are intimately connected, and Frankenstein and the creature are both simultaneously suffering hero and tormenting monster.

as if he is aiming a bow and arrow, but the weapon is not depicted. The painting was left unfinished though an earlier pen study for the work does show the hunting implements.

The starring role in the painting is given to the eagle. Fuseli has depicted the bird as a near dragon-type monster, with bright red eyes. The eagle's dark wings shroud almost the entire right side of the painting in darkness. The bird bends over the body of Prometheus in a possessive way, and threateningly raises its head at Herakles, like a predator protecting its prey in a nature documentary. Here we see the aforementioned fascination with the monstrous and macabre, typical in romantic art, exemplified in a way that was unimaginable to neoclassical artists.

A PROMETHEUS LANDSCAPE

The romantic theme of the depiction of the sublime, or the might of nature, can also be found in Promethean iconography. A poignant example of this is a work from 1847 by the American landscape painter Thomas Cole (1801-1848) (fig. 11.5). Cole was born in England but lived and worked in the United States. In the early years after the American Revolutionary War and subsequent establishment of the United States, there wasn't much time or money available to invest in art. This started to change in the early nineteenth century, as America started to look for its own artistic identity—something that could set it apart culturally from the old world that it had distanced itself from. This identity was finally found in the American landscape, the vastness of which starkly contrasted with the rapidly urbanising and densely-populated Europe.

In 1847, Cole submitted his *Prometheus Bound* to an art competition for works that were to adorn the Houses of Parliament in London. The work wasn't so much a history piece depicting the myth of Prometheus as it was a 'Prometheus landscape.' Before anything else, it is a depiction of an impressive, yet serene, mountainous landscape, bathed in morning light. Prometheus is present in the composition, but he can almost be overlooked, as he is completely overshadowed by the rocks. The viewer is startled by his appearance: eyes wandering over the serene peaks, we are suddenly faced with the

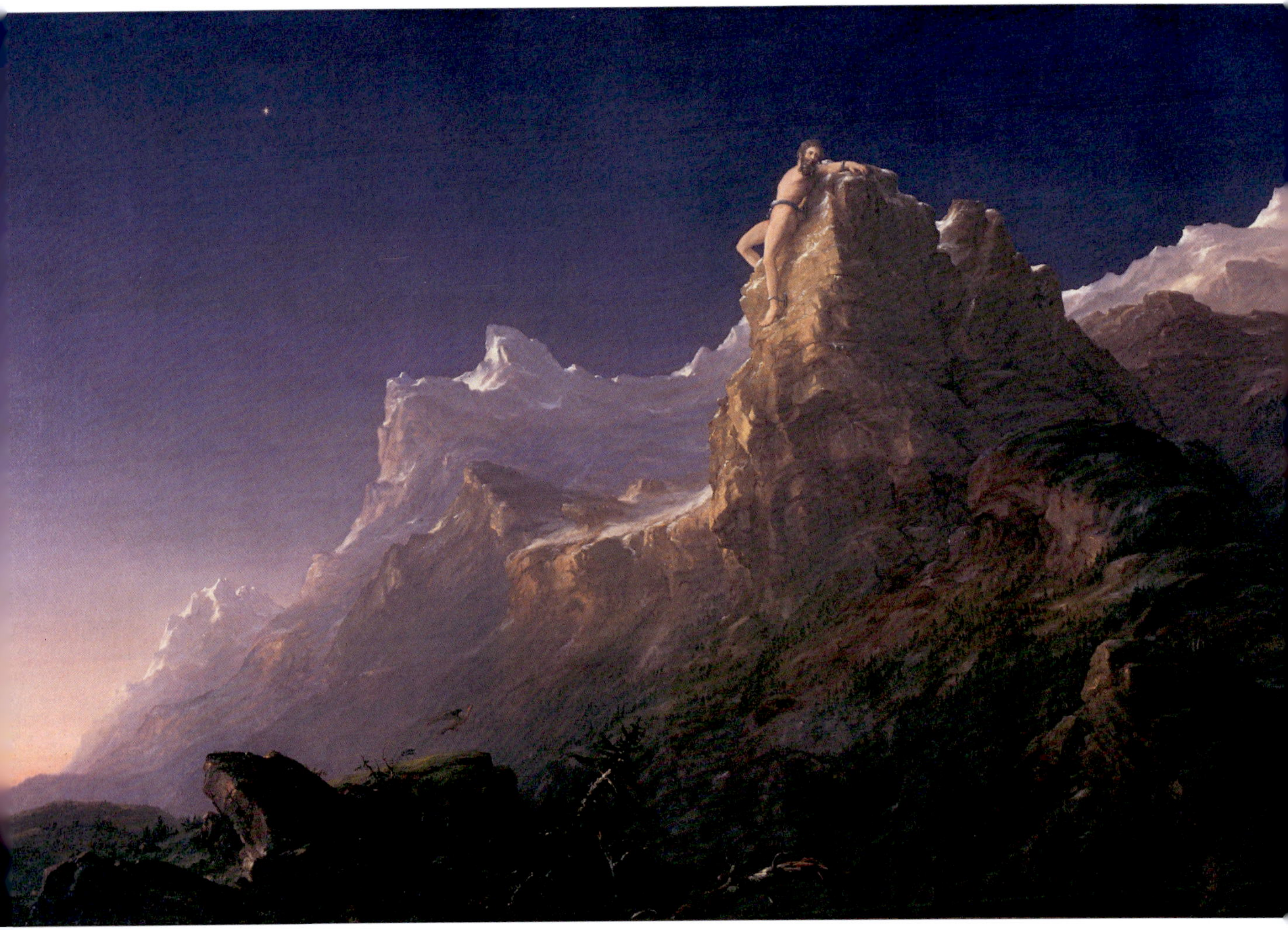

Titan's tortured body. The extent of the punishment is implied. From the forested valley, a vulture ascends towards Prometheus, the Morningstar, Jupiter, shines in the heavens. Cole wrote that he had purposely chosen to replace the eagle with a vulture, because he couldn't make the national bird of the United States commit such a horrible act. He also elucidated that the 'morning star' is the planet Jupiter; the watchful eye of Zeus (Jupiter) observes the fulfilment of his judgement in the guise of the 'morning star.' Cole chose the morning as the moment of punishment because the morning was the time of day that people felt the greatest amount of hope. But, for Prometheus, it was the time of his greatest despair. Perhaps Cole had succeeded too well in making a quintessentially American work, because it was poorly received in England and it both lost the contest and failed to sell. Finally, it had to be transported back to the United States.

Fig. 11.5 Thomas Cole, mountainscape / Prometheus bound to the Caucasus, 1847, oil paint on canvas, 162 x 243 cm, Fine Arts Museum of San Francisco, San Francisco

Cole's painting has truly gigantic dimensions that only further emphasize the expansiveness of the landscape. This makes it easy to overlook a salient detail. Prometheus is honouring his titanic nature with his size; he has the size of an entire mountain-top. In previous depictions of the Titan, Prometheus was always depicted on a human scale; he was not any larger than the trees or other figures that surrounded him. Yet, despite his monumental size, the grandeur of the landscape still dwarves him, emphasizing his vulnerability and perhaps even his humanity.

The myth of Prometheus was a politically charged subject in the 1840s in the United States. Prometheus was associated with rebellion against tyranny and in that guise, he was used as a symbol for the abolition of slavery. A poignant example of this is found in a poem by the poet and abolitionist James Russell Lowell (1819-1891). Lowell called Prometheus, 'the Locofoco of Greek mythology.' The Locofocos were a faction of the Democratic Party that strongly propagated the abolitionist cause. During a meeting of this group, their opponents decided to hinder them by cutting off the gas supply of the lamps in their meeting hall. Those congregated, however, had a large supply of 'Loco-foco' with them, a type of self-lighting cigar which turned into a match type and company, which they used to create makeshift torches, and continued their meeting. This event

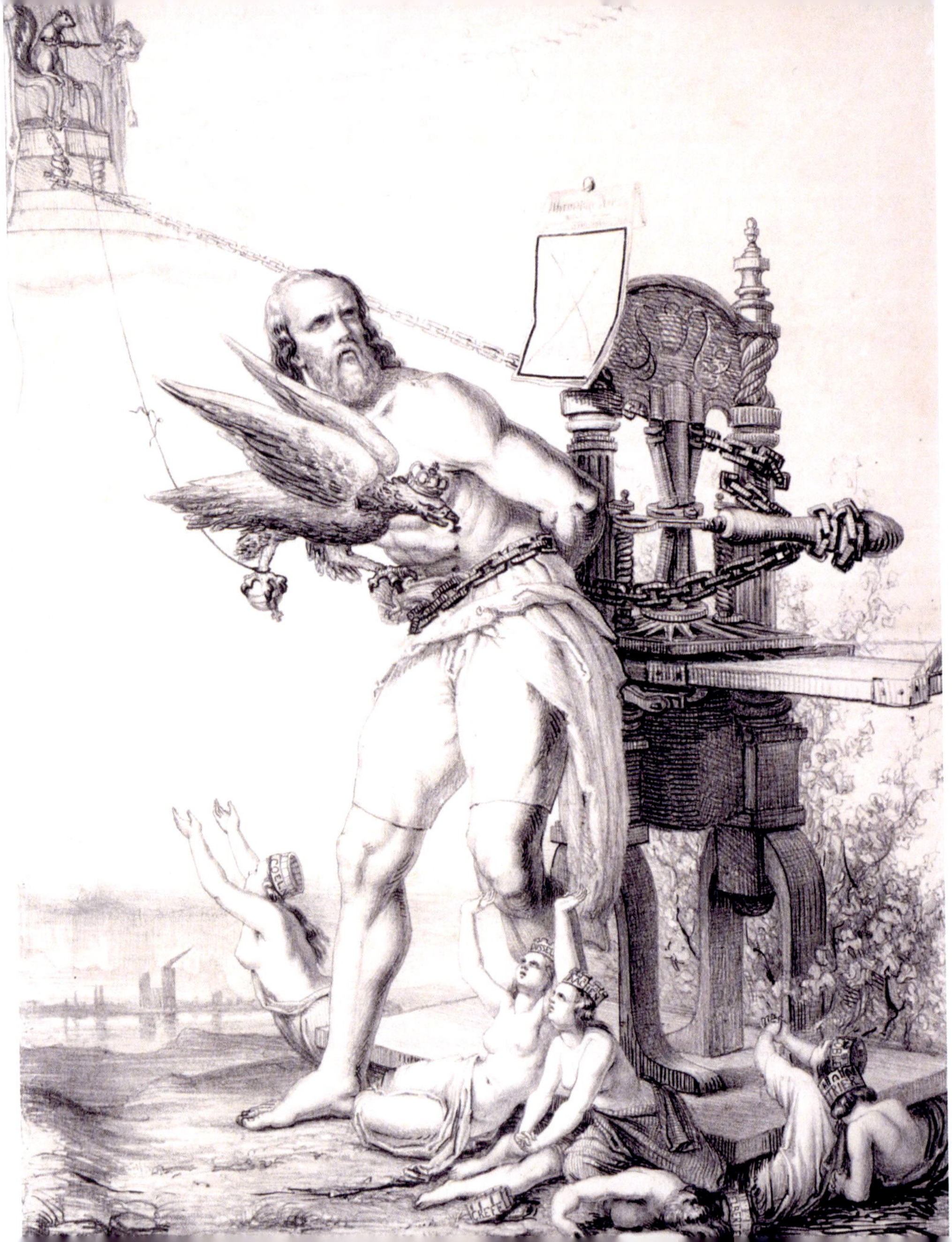

Fig. 11.6 Lorenz Clasen, Karl Marx in the guise of Prometheus chained to a silenced printing press. Minister 'Eichhorn' (squirrel) sends the Prussian eagle to torment him. The caricature was made because of the ban on the Rheinische Zeitung. 843, lithograph, 46,5 x 31 cm, Deutsches Historisches Museum, Berlin

gained them the nickname, 'Locofocos.' Such torchbearers, who oppose tyranny and oppression, were thus very appropriately compared to Prometheus in Lowell's poem.

Thomas Cole never explicitly confirmed or denied that his *Prometheus Bound* contained a similar political message. He did, however, make other landscapes that contained political messages, an example of which would be his *The Course of Empire* series, which points to empire as a possible source of decay of civilisation. Given the political climate in which he produced his work, it is possible that Cole's Prometheus landscape references a subtle and poetic abolitionist message.

THE POLITICAL PROMETHEUS

A more explicit usage of the Prometheus figure to deliver political commentary can be found in a caricature by Lorenz Clasen (1812-1899) from 1843 (fig. 11.6). In the image, we see Karl Marx depicted as Prometheus chained to a printing press. Prometheus was Marx's favourite mythological figure and the philosopher turned to the Titan on multiple occasions to create metaphors in his philosophy. To Marx, Prometheus represented reason that rebelled against the restraints cast upon progress by religion. In his renowned book *Das Kapital*, Marx compared Prometheus to the proletariat that is chained by capital. His anti-religious and anti-capitalist philosophy was deemed dangerous by the people in power around him; in 1843, the *Rheinische Zeitung*, of which Marx was editor, was forbidden to be published by Karl Friedrich Eichhorn, Prussian minister of religious and educational affairs. This event prompted Lorenz Clasen to make his caricature, where he criticised the minister's censorship.

In the upper-left corner of the image, we see a small squirrel on a throne—a play on the minister's last name (Eichhörnchen is squirrel in German)—who is literally holding the reigns, controlling the rest of the scene. The chains with which Marx—in the role of Prometheus—is chained to the broken printing press are attached to the legs of the throne. The squirrel is controlling the eagle as if he is flying a kite and has the bird peck into Marx's left side. This is not the side of the body where the liver is situated. This reversal could once again be the result of the mirroring effect that the engraving technique has, but since all text in the image is not reversed it could also be a visual pun that Marx is tormented on his left side, referencing his leftist ideology. The eagle is wearing a little crown and is holding the emperor's orb, clearly referencing the Prussian eagle. By Marx's feet sit personifications of the cities of the Rhineland, bemoaning the loss of the journal as the Oceanids who, in Aeschylus' tragedy, mourn the fate of Prometheus. The crowns on the heads of these cities personified signify which towns they each represent.

PROMETHEUS AND SYMBOLISM, LOOKING FOR A LOST CONNECTION

In the second half of the nineteenth century, an art movement emerged that sought to represent truths as symbols, using metaphor to relate ideals. This movement, aptly named Symbolism, was an expansion on Romantic stylistic tendencies, showing many similarities with the earlier period. The discontent with the long-term effects of progress-minded attitudes and rationalism, as well as a sense of loss after revolution upon revolution, both political and scientific, only grew stronger as the century progressed. A good deal of the new art movements that this period produced were rationalistic in nature. For example, impressionism and realism both sought to represent the world as it truly was. Realism did this through its choice of subject matter: no longer should one paint lofty biblical or mythological scenes, but instead depict poor workers. Impressionism attempted to achieve this through artistic technique: inspired by new developments in optics, it set out to capture a fleeting moment through suggestion of light and colour.

Symbolism served as a counter-reaction to this matter-of-fact rationalism. It set out to depict not the material world, but rather the immaterial truth behind it. According to the symbolists, church, state, art and language were all instances of sets of symbols that reflected a deeper inner hidden truth, an absolute ideal. The symbolists believed that the focus of other art movements on material reality, paired with the loss of these old structures of meaning, caused a loss of connection with that deeper truth. They sought

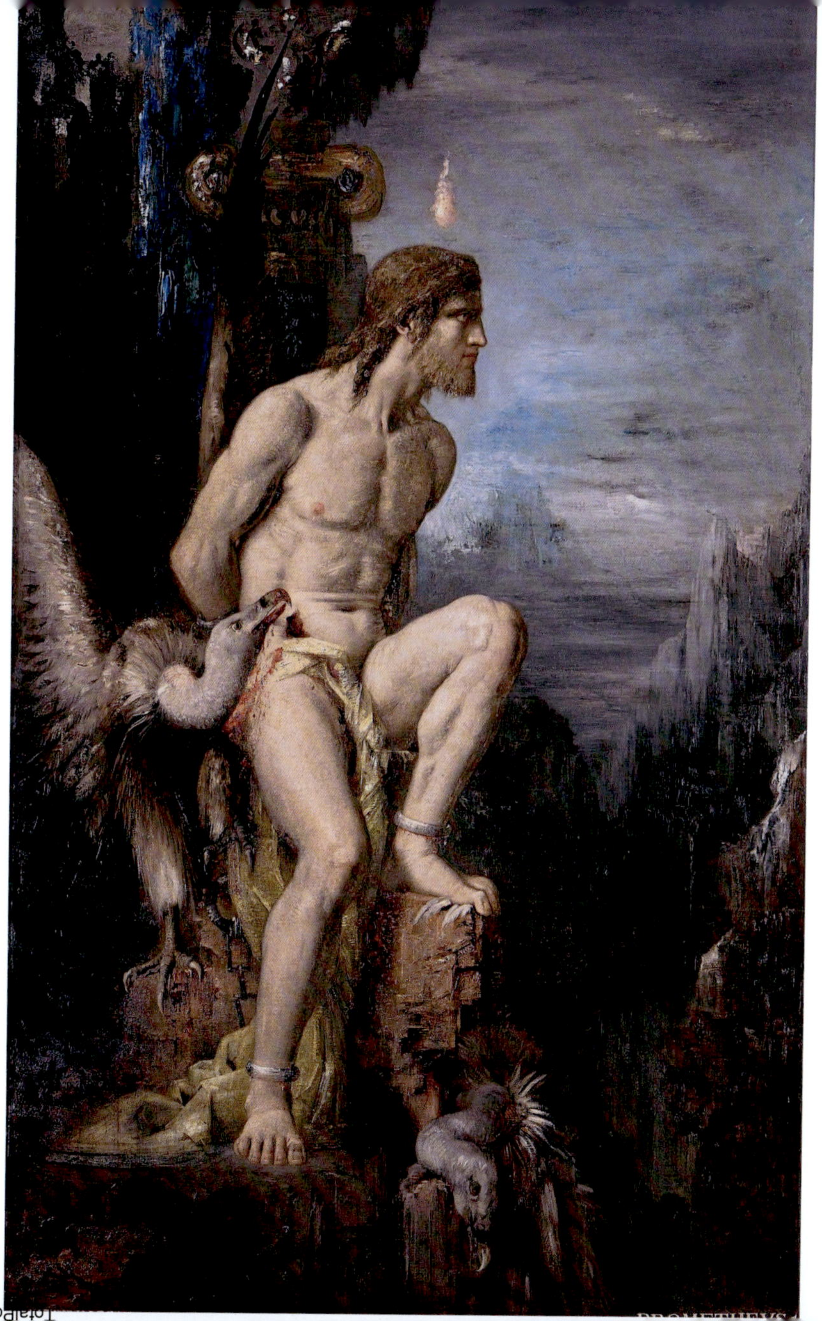

Fig. 11.7 Gustave Moreau, Promethée, the hero is chained to a column on the Caucasus. The hero looks forward, seemingly undisturbed while a vulture pecks into his side. A second vulture lies dead at his feet. Above the head of Prometheus floats a mysterious wisp of fire. 1868, Oil paint on Canvas, 205 x 122 cm, Musée Gustave Moreau, Paris

to reconnect to this deeper truth by utilising mystical, dreamlike imagery. To fulfil that purpose, they often used figures from classical mythology. These figures were not used in the traditional, strictly iconographic sense, where there is a unilateral reference to antiquity, but rather in a highly personalised and ambiguous way, in order to express that part of the hidden ideal the myth reflected according to their interpretations.

The French painter Gustave Moreau (1826-1898) was one of the most prolific artists of the Symbolist movement. He was fascinated by the potential of Prometheus as a symbol and turned to the Titan as subject multiple times in his work. For Moreau, Prometheus stood for the human struggle that emerges when idealism clashes with realism and the subsequent misunderstanding that follows from this clash. Moreau's most well-known painting of the Titan, *Promethée*, which he made in 1868, was displayed at the Salon of Paris in 1869 (fig. 11.7). In the image, Moreau paints Prometheus in a yet unseen manner. Instead of suffering through his punishment, Prometheus seems indifferent to it and stares ahead in an unaffected manner; this is a clear reference to the translation of his name as 'he who looks ahead.' He is depicted sitting amidst a mountainous landscape, chained to a column, as described by Hesiod. Moreau did take liberties with the literary source material; the punishment is not executed by an eagle but instead by two vultures, which originally were assigned to Tityus. Prometheus seems to be ignoring the vulture that has pecked a gash into his side and still has the Titan's flesh in its beak. It is remarkable that the wound is positioned rather low on the stomach, instead of in its more typical position just under the ribs, as we have seen in the baroque depictions of the Titan's punishment. The second vulture lies dead at the feet of Prometheus, a reference to his eventual triumph and liberation at the hand of Herakles.

The most remarkable attribute of the piece, however, is the strong resemblance between Prometheus and Christ. Prometheus' appearance, with shoulder-length, brown and wavy hair, as well as his beard are reminiscent of traditional western depictions of Christ. An even more explicit reference to Christ is the little flame hovering above Prometheus' head. In Christian iconography, such a flame in this location denotes a person who has been 'illuminated' by the Holy Ghost; it is, for example, traditionally depicted above the heads of Christ's followers at Pentecost. Moreau seems to want to suggest with this detail that Prometheus is an enlightened spirit in kind, equally illuminated by the 'fire of reason' that he stole from the gods. It is likely that Moreau intended this flame to be read as a Christian motif. In an earlier study for this painting, Moreau had crowned Prometheus with a halo – unmistakably 'Christianising' him.

This intermingling of Christian and pagan symbolism shows just how the Symbolists approached their subjects: the symbols they used did not reference one clear and decipherable source or meaning, as had been the case with the allegories of the Renaissance. According to Moreau, both Christ and Prometheus were symbols of the same absolute principle due to the sacrifices they made. This principle is the human struggle with idealism (the divine fire of Prometheus, and the divine word of Christ), which collides with materialism and lack of understanding resulting in their torment. Because the two figures as symbols referenced the same underlying subconscious principle and, through that principle, express the spiritual experiences of the artist, they could be used almost interchangeably, their iconography and narrative becoming intermingled.

This strongly individualistic approach of the myth by symbolist painters is a phenomenon that only expanded in the twentieth century. In the previous chapters, Prometheus has been discussed in light of a single and chronological artistic current or development. In the twentieth century, art movements started succeeding each other so rapidly that the lens with which to view the myth is no longer so clear. Instead, the relationship between individual artists and Prometheus will be brought to the forefront of discourse on the Titan in twentieth-century art making, discussed in chapter thirteen.

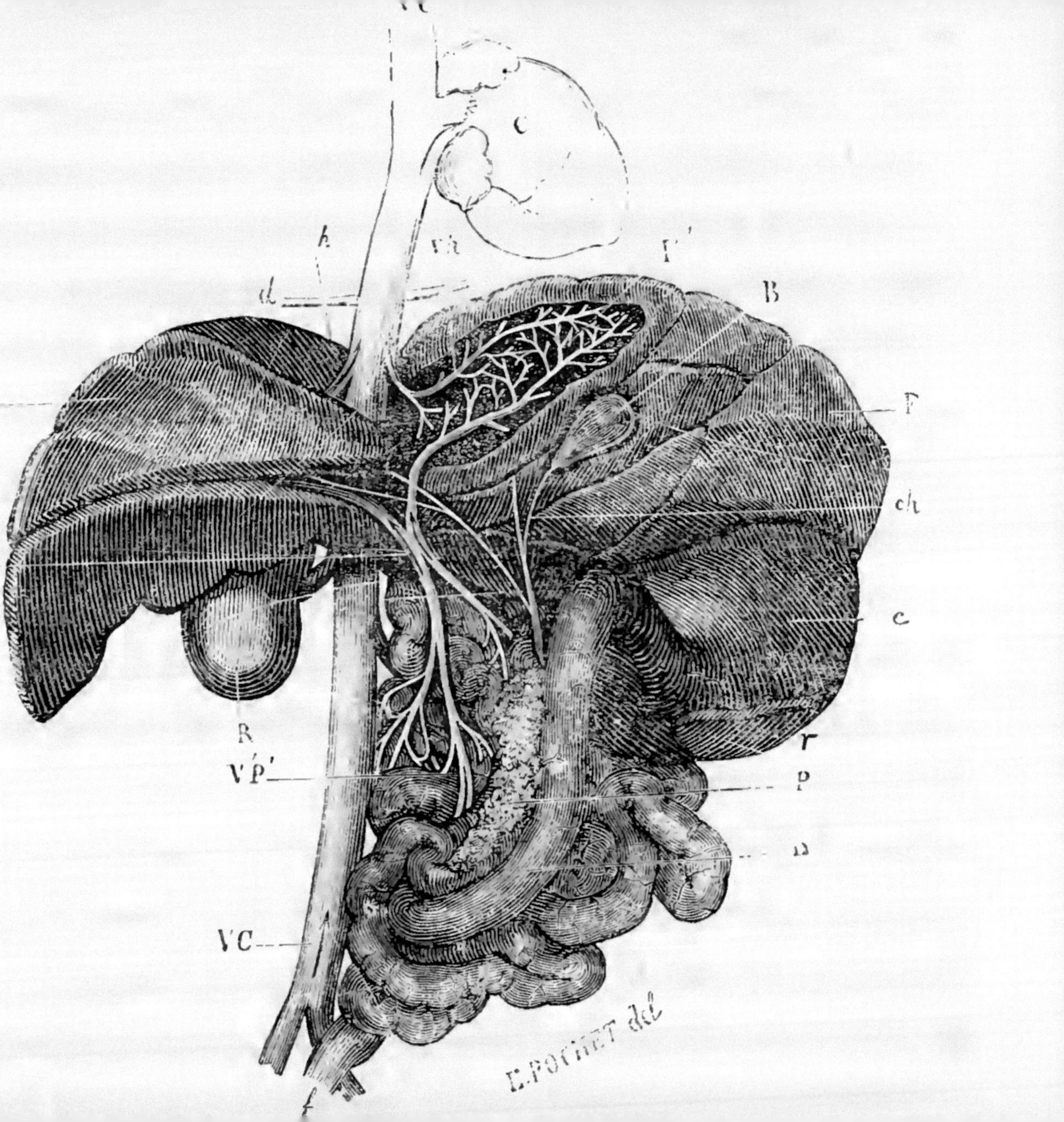

h
vh
d
C
F'
B
F
F
VP
ch
c
R
r
V'P'
p
VC
E. POCHET del

12
THE LIVER IN THE ENLIGHTENMENT

ALBRECHT VON HALLER, FOUNDATIONAL THINKER OF THE PHYSIOLOGY OF THE LIVER

One of the most important scientists of the eighteenth century, often called the last 'homo universalis' of his time, was the Swiss doctor Albrecht von Haller (1708-1777, Fig. 12.1). He wasn't solely a famed doctor, anatomist, surgeon and physiologist, but he also made a name for himself as a botanist and poet. He was the son of a lawyer from Bern and showed signs of being a prodigy from a very young age. At only nine years old, he composed a Hebrew and Greek dictionary from words

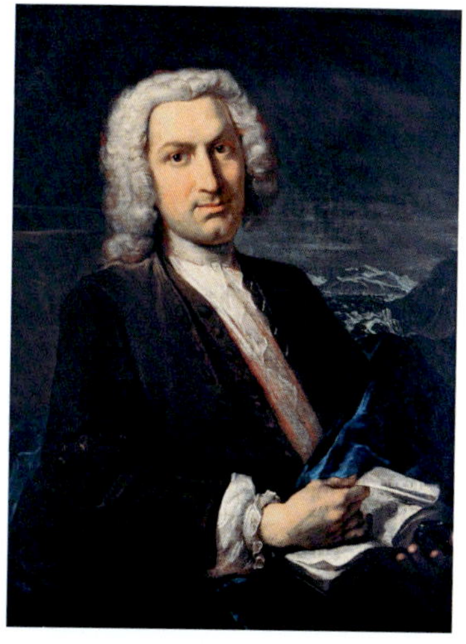

Fig. 12.1 Johann Rudolf Huber, portrait of Albrecht von Haller, 1736

Fig. 12.0 Internal image of the liver to illustrate the process of sugar metabolism. The blood that is supplied from the intestines flows into the liver through the portal vein and its branches. In the liver tissue, sugar is transformed into glucose which is then taken up into the blood again. Through the draining veins of the liver, the blood flows into the caval vein (vena cava inferior) *of the abdomen. From: Claude Bernard,* Leçons de physiologie expérimentale appliquée à la médecine, faites au Collège de France, *tome I, Baillière, Paris, 1855*

that he had managed to glean from the Bible. At the same age, he also wrote two thousand short biographies of notable figures from history. When he was fifteen years old, Albrecht von Haller started his medical studies in Tübingen, where he soon deemed the quality of education to be subpar. He decided to continue his studies in Leiden, inspired by Professor Herman Boerhaave, famed all throughout Europe, whose study books Haller had read. At the university of Leiden, the promising young student experienced a golden age. With permission from Boerhaave, he committed himself to his botanical studies in the botanical gardens of the university and, under the supervision of the anatomist Bernard Siegfried Albinus Jr., he was allowed to partake in anatomical dissections on cadavers. He obtained a doctorate in 1727 in Leiden, writing his dissertation on the ducts of the salivary gland.

After visiting London, Paris, Basel and Bern, Haller – by now a renowned scientist – was made professor in medicine, anatomy, botany and surgery at the University of Göttingen. He established a *theatrum anatomicum* there, which he utilised for his physiological experiments, and founded his own botanical garden. Haller wrote his *Elementa physiologiae corporis humani* in Göttingen, the first systematic treatise on the physiology of the human body. It is a monumental work consisting of eight volumes that appeared over the course of 1757-1766. The knowledge of physiology that he displayed in this voluminous work would dominate medical practice in the eighteenth century and well into the nineteenth century.

The sixth part of Haller's magnum opus is dedicated to the anatomy and function of the liver. In this part, he summarised everything that had been discovered about the liver up to his day and supplied his own critical annotations and findings. He greatly valued the use of experiment and direct observation, and was able to prove his theories with empirical data. With his study book, Haller laid the foundation for hepatology—the field of study dedicated to the treatment of liver diseases—as we know it today.

Three out of the only six anatomical plates in Haller's eight-part corpus depict the anatomy of the liver (fig. 12.2). They show the organ and the course of the bile ducts and blood vessels with a level of detail not inferior to our contemporary anatomical depictions of this organ.

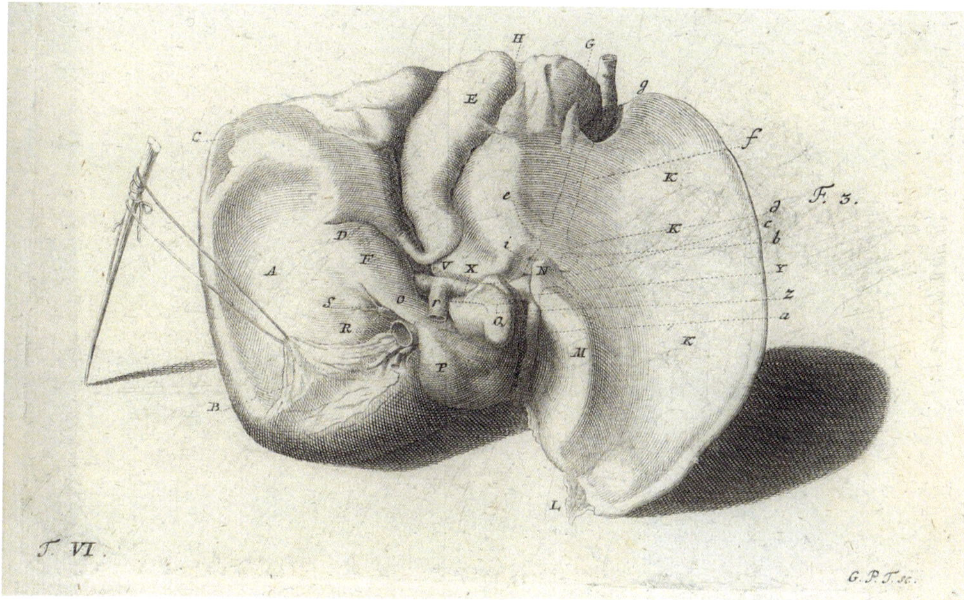

Fig. 12.2 Engraving from Haller's study book Elementa physiologiae corporis humani *(1757-1766). Depicted is the underside of the liver with the anatomical right lobe (A), left lobe (K), and gallbladder (E)*

Haller suspected that the liver had a far more vital function than had been previously assumed. The common opinion was that it served for the production of blood, given the deep red colour of the organ (which, as we now know, is caused by the dense network of small blood vessels in liver tissue). The bile was seen solely as excrement that was collected in the liver and was used to expel waste products. Haller, on the other hand, reasoned that it couldn't possibly be the case that the sole purpose of the largest organ in the abdominal cavity was to carry off a byproduct like bile. In addition to this reasoning, he knew—by dissecting human and animal cadavers—that the bile duct is connected to the duodenum, right after the stomach (fig. 12.3). According to Haller, this would indicate that bile served a specific purpose in the digestive process in the intestinal tract.

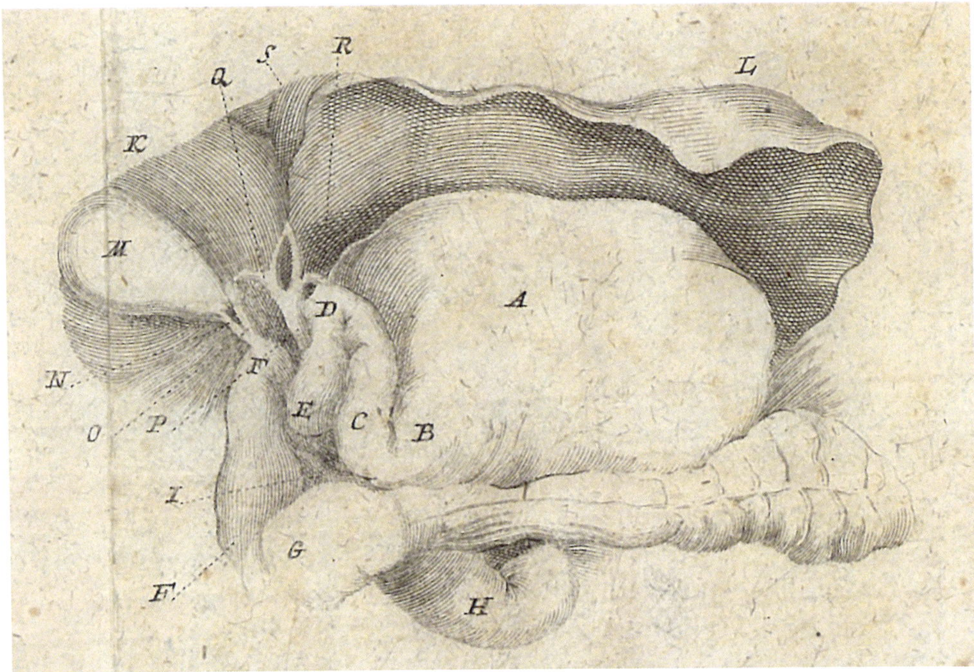

Fig. 12.3 The gallbladder secretes bile into the duodenum (D/E). The bile from the gallbladder flows through a branch (N) that leads to the bile duct (O). Engraving of the liver from Haller's textbook Elementa physiologiae corporis humani

Haller described bile as a slippery, soap-like substance that would serve to help break down excess fats in food, so it could be better absorbed into the body. By tying off the bile duct in animals, Haller was able to show that this would lead to a stagnation of bile, which resulted in jaundice. Haller postulated that gallstones could block the bile duct in a similar manner, which would lead to a wide variety of digestive issues and pain, with a yellow discoloration of the entire body as an end result—all due to the congestion of bile. Hence, he demonstrated the interrelation between obstruction of the bile duct and the occurrence of jaundice.

CLAUDE BERNARD, DISCOVERER OF THE SUGAR METABOLISM IN THE LIVER

By the end of the eighteenth century, the external anatomy of the liver was well defined and attention shifted to the internal workings of the liver, in compliance with the new modernised scientific approach of that time. After Haller had laid the scientific foundations for physiology, scientists at the onset of the nineteenth century further researched the function of the liver, partially informed by new insights provided by the chemical-physiological sciences.

The physiologist Claude Bernard (1813-1878) is one of the people who provided a fundamental contribution to the understanding of the liver, especially concerning the metabolism that takes place during the process of digestion. Bernard studied medicine in Paris and afterwards dedicated himself fully to experimental research in the laboratory, for which a special chair at the Sorbonne University was created. He discovered that the liver contains glucose and that the levels of glucose in the liver were regulated by the storage of sugar in the liver by the levels of glycogen. As it had been known for centuries that the liver produced the excretion of bile, Bernard was the first in a long time to demonstrate a new function of the liver: the internal secretion of glucose. His goal was to use his experimental research to bridge a gap between physiology and research into the origin and treatment of diseases. With his work that transgressed the discipline's boundaries, he made the first strides into what would become modern liver physiology.

By this time, towards the end of the nineteenth century, the association of Prometheus and the myth loosened, while Prometheus in arts and literature served as a symbol, the rebel challenging power and oppression. Less emphasis was therefore, placed on the liver that had been tormented by the eagle and represented Prometheus's main suffering. In medical science, interest in the liver and its intricacies continued and it was in the spirit of Prometheus that the scientific limits of that time were challenged too, enlighting the liver in all its aspects.

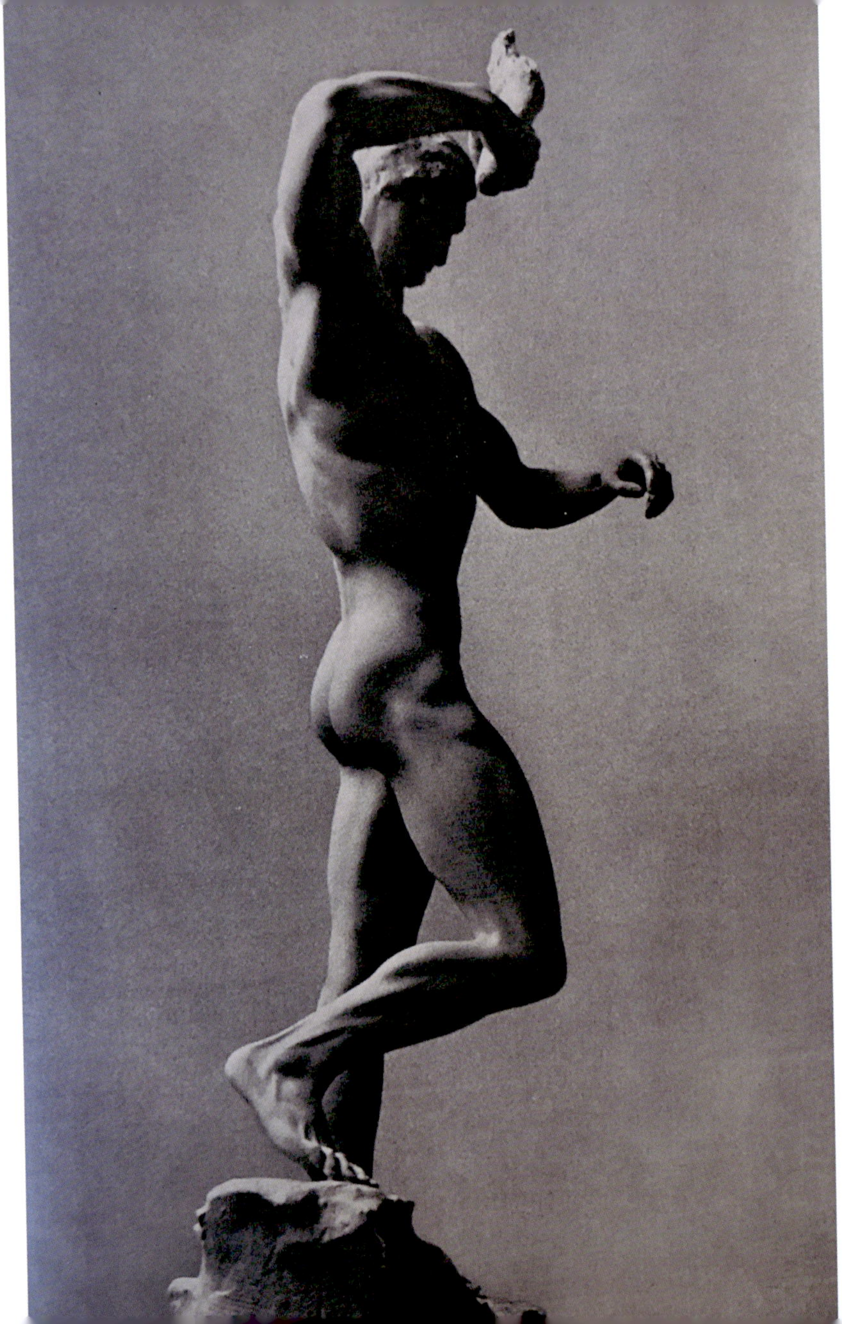

13 THE TWENTIETH-CENTURY PROMETHEUS

At the end of our chapter on modernity (chapter eleven), we discussed how artists began to approach the subject of Prometheus in increasingly individualistic ways. Instead of referencing a classical source, Prometheus became a vehicle through which artists could express personal convictions. This relationship was solidified in the twentieth century, a period in which art movements followed one another in rapid succession: expressionism, futurism, cubism, etc. The century is sometimes affectionately called the 'time of the many '-isms." The twentieth century was also shaped by two world wars, the effects of which greatly impacted philosophical and artistic thought. In this chapter, we will show how artists utilised the Prometheus myth to frame their own individual artistic ideologies.

Fig. 13.0 Arno Brecker, Prometheus descends from the Olympus with the fire for humanity. 1934, Bronze, Museum Arno Breker/MARCO-VG, Bonn

LOOKING AHEAD AND BEING AHEAD OF THE CURVE: KUPKA'S AVANT-GARDE PROMETHEUS

At the onset of the twentieth century, a variety of avant-garde art movements emerged that experimented with style in yet unprecedented ways. Many artists turned away from the concept that art always had to correspond with the empirical truth. Instead, they

Fig. 13.1 František Kupka, the red-blue Prometheus. Prometheus is depicted nude and heroic. His head is crowned by a halo of hair and he clutches a fennel stalk like a sceptre. 1909-1910, watercolours, 321 x 293 mm, National Gallery, Prague

each developed their own aesthetic identity, rejecting the notion of one universal mode of perception. This departure from realism opened the road towards abstraction. František Kupka (1871-1957) was one painter working at the time of this juncture. Kupka was, for some time, associated with the Vienna Secession, a symbolist movement that earned its name for its departure from the artistic establishment—Gustav Klimt was one of its most prolific members. The art produced by this movement was typified by the use of repetitive geometrical motifs.

This can be seen quite clearly in František Kupka's *Prometheus* (fig. 13.1). We are faced with a fully nude Prometheus, who stands proudly, surrounded by nature. His head is haloed by the curls of his hair, which resemble solar rays. These curls in his hair and indeed the stylized, almost quivering rays of summer heat that frame the figure, form the geometrical patterns that are so typical of the Secession movement. Kupka was also influenced by the French avant-garde who, in rejection of modernity, found inspiration in what they reductively deemed 'primitive' forms of art, the most well-known example being Picasso's fascination with African masks. František Kupka, in turn, found his greatest inspiration in ancient Etruscan and Babylonian art. The fierce stature and muscular chest of Prometheus, even the way he holds his fennel stalk like a sceptre, are indeed reminiscent of Gilgamesh or depictions of Babylonian kings. Kupka utilised line and colour freely to express his personal emotions and spirituality, intimately connected to the philosophy he subscribed to: orphism. Orphism promotes the idea that cosmic order and the laws of nature are incarnated in humans. According to the practitioners of orphism, humans are nature made self-aware, and thus able to rise above primordial chaos. For Kupka, Prometheus signified the end of the era of supreme reign of the primordial Olympic nature gods, and signified the start of the era of man.

Over the course of his career, František Kupka turned away from figurative art and towards abstraction, becoming one of the pioneers of abstract art. However, Kupka did not produce an abstract Prometheus. This was eventually completed by a different pioneer of abstraction: the sculptor Constantin Brâncuşi (1876-1957).

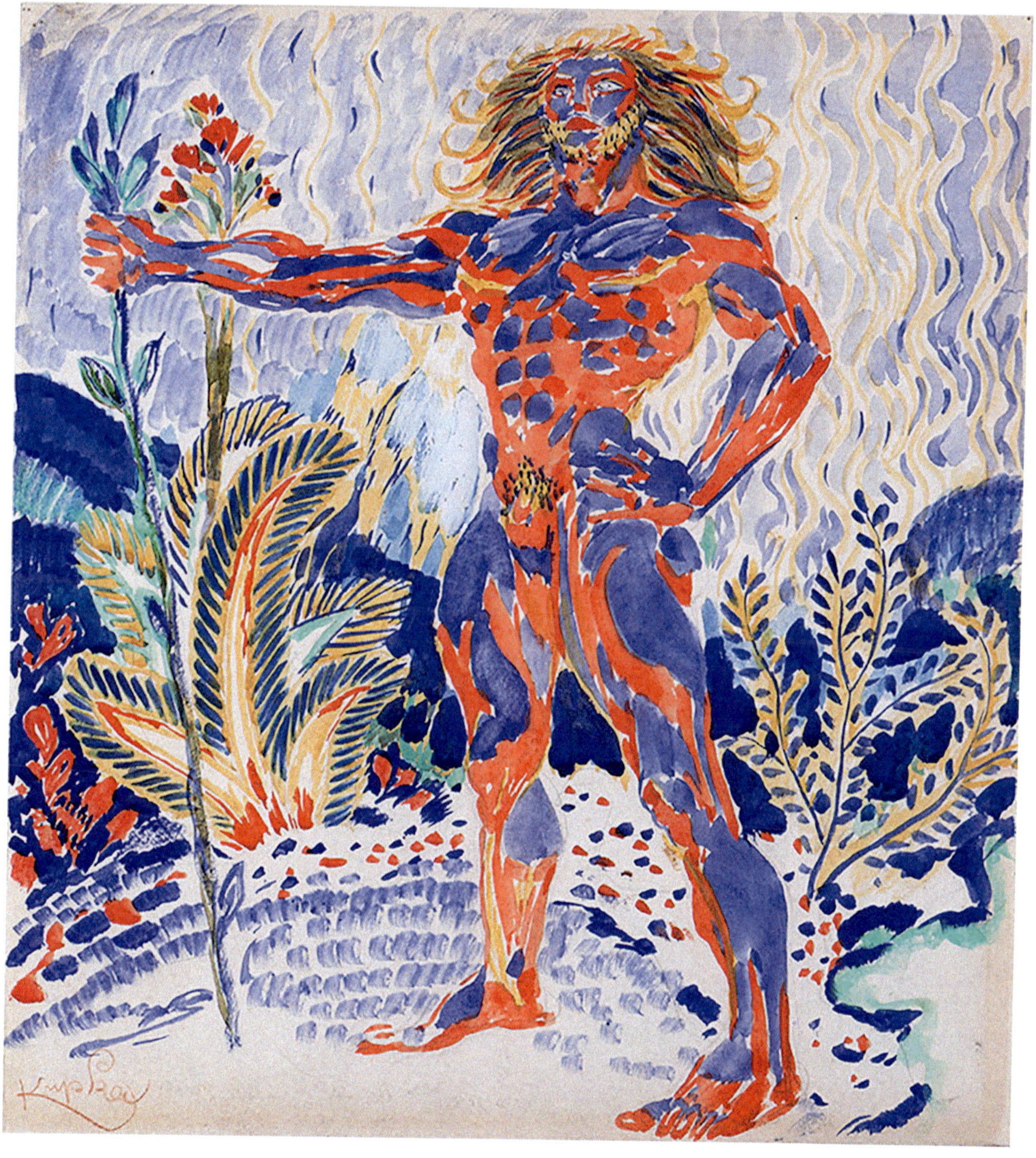

THE ABSTRACT ESSENCE OF PROMETHEUS

Brâncuşi was born far removed from the 'modernity' that consumed Europe's big cities. Growing up in a remote Romanian village called Hobița, Brâncuşi was instructed in the local folkloric art tradition of sculpture. After completing his education, he moved to Paris, where worked as an assistant to the avant-garde sculptor Rodin for a while. Brâncuşi was quick to emancipate himself from the great master, eager to step out of Rodin's shadow, and radically turned away from the sculpting tradition that preceded him. In his sculptures, Brâncuşi sought to depict the pure essence of his subjects. He stripped away any and all unnecessary details until he reached what he called a 'geometrical truth,' located within the most basic shape that remained after carving.

Fig. 13.2 Constantin Brancussi, Prometheus. 1911, white marble, 13,7 × 17,8 × 13,7 cm, Philadelphia Museum of Art, Philadelphia

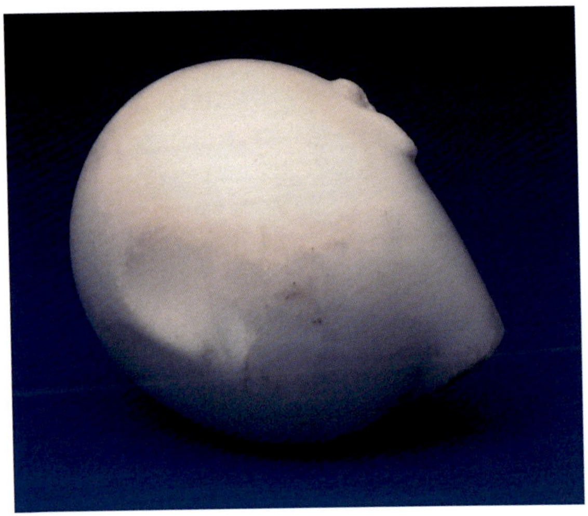

The artist was fascinated by birds and their flight, and they make up an important part of his oeuvre. However, when he decided to depict Prometheus, the 'absolute essence' of the myth to him was not located in the eagle, but in the head of the hero (fig. 13.2). Brâncuşi's Prometheus is simply the Titan's head, oriented on its side, the face turned down to the surface it is placed upon. In this pose, it resembles the rocks of the Caucasus Mountains. A small protrusion at the top suggests an ear, and under that we find the arc of the eyebrow and a nose. By working with these kinds of 'reduced' depictions of his subjects, Brâncuşi had the opportunity to give more attention to other aspects of the works. He seems to have given great consideration to how his works might interact with their environment, the influence of the pedestal, the material, and the spectator experience of the artwork. In the case of this sculpture of Prometheus, Brâncuşi mostly experimented with the expressiveness of the material. In addition to this first iteration in marble, Brâncuşi made the same sculpture in gilded bronze, gypsum and rock.

The time in which Kupka and Brâncuşi worked was characterised by a blind faith in modernity on one side – that is to say, of faith in the myth of linear progress in the development in history – and the imminent looming threat of rising political tensions on the world stage that that would eventually result in the first world war, on the other. The devastation brought on by this war would bring the idealism and modernist ideals of progress to a grinding halt, which is reflected in the type of art produced during and after the two world wars.

A GOLDEN PROMETHEUS: ROCKEFELLER'S AMERICAN DREAM

In the United States, far removed from the grim reality of war and on the other side of the ocean, modern art was slower to gain a foothold; here, the dream of progress was alive and well. We encountered an example of the search for an American artistic identity—a style suited to tell the American story—in Thomas Cole's *Prometheus Landscape*, discussed in chapter eleven of this book (fig. 11.4). The use of Prometheus to tell the American story reaches its peak in the statue of the Titan that adorns the Rockefeller Center in New York City.

J.D. Rockefeller (1874-1960) was a rich philanthropist who, in the early 1930s, commissioned a large building complex that would contain offices and stores. He leased the ground on which the complex was built he from Columbia University. Rockefeller took a large financial risk when building the complex, as the United States was in the throes of great economic depression. Despite the private nature of the building project, it received support from the so-called 'City Beautiful Movement.' This movement promoted large-scale urban planning projects that benefitted the population. The aim was to elevate American cities to a higher level so they could rival their European predecessors. So, the City Beautiful Movement adorned American cities with boulevards and promenades, favouring a neoclassical style and seeking to create American equivalents of the Athenian Acropolis or the Roman forum.

The Rockefeller Center consists of several art deco skyscrapers interspersed with large, open lines of sight to form a visual axis, creating something akin to European boulevards. The complex contained enough open space for the public that it attracted the interests of the City Beautiful Movement, who facilitated an integrated art program. The walkway boulevard leading up to the central skyscraper was dubbed the mythological alley, filled with fountains containing tritons and Nereids (sea nymphs). The shining crown of this boulevard is a monumental fountain containing a statue of Prometheus stealing the fire (fig. 13.3).

This Prometheus embodies the central values that Rockefeller envisioned to be associated with his complex: the virtues that drive humanity forward. Prometheus represented the coming together of these virtues: he possessed determination, leadership, cool, rational thinking, unbridled energy and the courage to take risks – all virtues that were in line with the American entrepreneurial spirit which, according to the City Beautiful Movement, would help America rival the Roman Empire in terms of grandeur. In this sense, Rockefeller also saw himself reflected in the hero; after all, he had taken the large financial risk to have the complex built during an economic crisis.

The Prometheus statue was created in 1934 by the sculptor Paul Manship. It is made out of gilded bronze, which brightly reflects sunlight and draws eyes to the end of the boulevard. The work is executed in a flowing, organic style, free from modernist or avant-garde experiments with form like the previous works discussed in this chapter. Prometheus is oriented in a unique horizontal position, but his proportions and anatomy are classical. He flies down on a zodiac ring, signifying that the fire he brings is celestial in nature. On the marble wall behind him we find a quotation after Aeschylus: 'Prometheus teacher in every art, brought the fire that hath proved to mortals a means to mighty ends.' The emphasis on Prometheus as benefactor of mankind was meant to reflect what Rockefeller as a philanthropist and his project could mean for New York. Prometheus was made to embody the 'American Dream.'

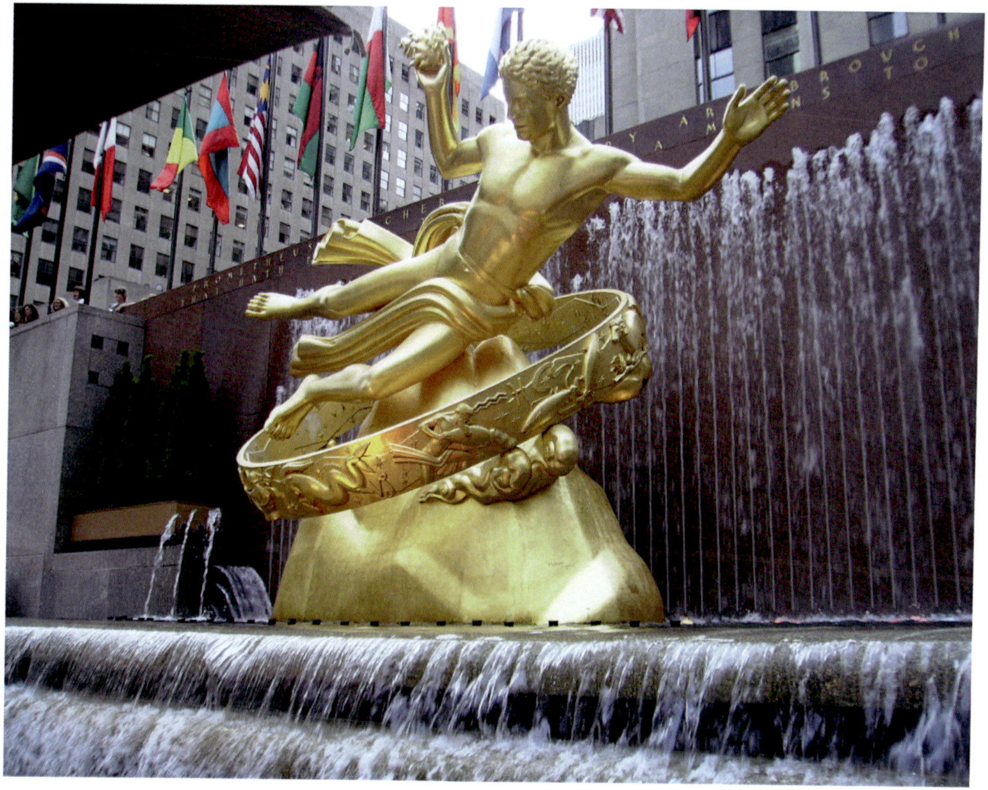

Fig. 13.3 Paul Manship, Prometheus fountain. Prometheus brings the heavenly fire to humanity, flying in on a zodiac ring. 1934, gilded bronze, 18,3 x 4,9 m, Rockefeller Centre, New York City

PROMETHEUS THE REVOLUTIONARY: OROZCO'S AMERICAN DREAM

During the same period, a different use of the Prometheus myth was developing in the United States that, in many ways, was opposite to Rockefeller's Prometheus. This contrary Prometheus can be located in a mural painted by the Mexican artist José Clemente Orozco (1883-1949) in Claremont, California (fig. 13.4). While Manship's creation used a conventional classical style, Orozco's style for his Prometheus was experimental and modernist. Where the Rockefeller statue reflected bourgeois values, the fresco in Claremont had a revolutionary character. Orozco's mural was commissioned by Pomona College to decorate their campus dining hall. Prometheus was a subject that seemed to fit the setting of a university: he was, after all, traditionally an example for scholars in that his act of bringing fire to humanity also brought reason. This was, however, only the superficial reading of the mural. Orozco was one of the most prominent artists of the

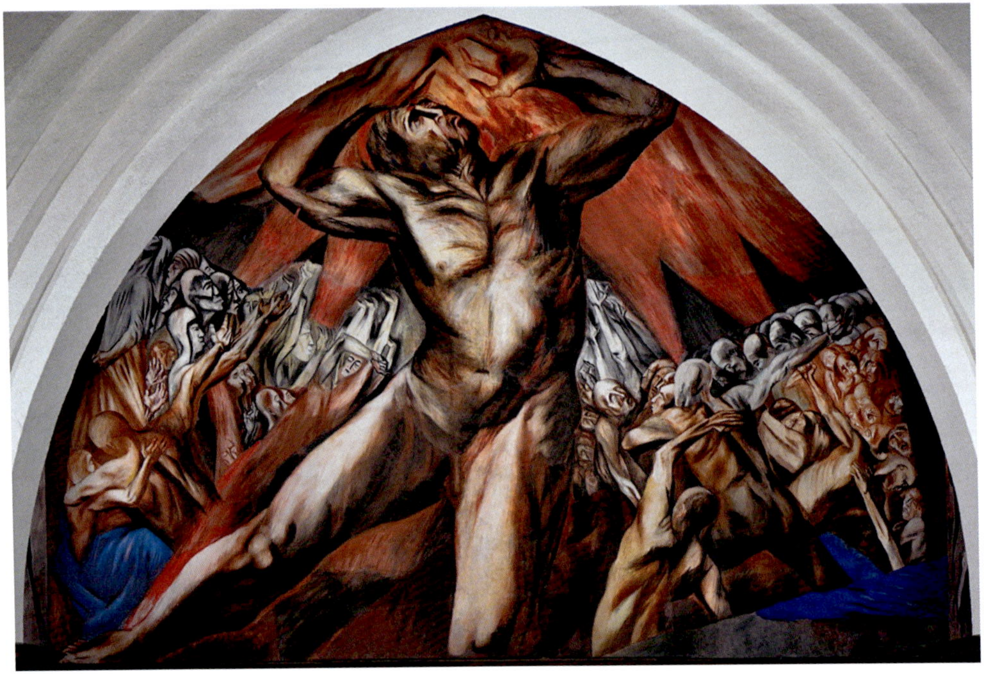

Fig. 13.4 José Clemente Orozco, Prometheus. Prometheus pulls down the divine fire with his bare hands. A large crowd of people has gathered around him, some extend their hands to him, while others turn away.1930, fresco in the dining hall of Pomona College, 610 × 870 m, Claremont CA

Mexican Muralism movement. This movement emerged from the Mexican Revolution, which took place between 1910 and 1920. Large, monumental murals containing political and socially critical messages were left in and on public buildings by the artists of this movement. Orozco had strong socialist sympathies and his work was generally critical of the toll the revolution took on the Mexican population and the violence that had accompanied it. When he made the Pomona College Prometheus, it was the first work by a member of the Mexican Muralism movement produced outside of Mexico and is often lauded as the first modernist wall painting in the United States.

Orozco's Prometheus bears a resemblance to the Titan's brother Atlas—who carried the heavens on his shoulders—in the way that Prometheus' hands reach for the ceiling. His outstretched hands grab the fire of heaven that pours out in red fiery beams over the crowds gathered by his feet. Orozco wrote in his commentary on the painting that he hoped to convey to viewers that this crowd was not a uniform mass, but rather a gathering of individuals that each have unique reactions to what is transpiring. Some of the figures turn away from Prometheus, shielding themselves, while others reach out towards the Titan and extend their hands to the fire. This is allegorical: progress, modernity and knowledge impact groups of people differently; some reap the benefits of it, but others bear the costs.

Prometheus also had great symbolical value for Orozco on a personal level, as a figure who rises up against oppression. The artist's journey to the United States knew many hardships: when crossing the border, border control agents destroyed all of the artworks he had brought with him. In addition to this loss, painting controversial topics posed a greater risk for him than it would to American citizens, as he could be arrested or deported if he was deemed a threat to public decency. For example, it is likely that Orozco depicted Prometheus without genitals in order to not offend American puritanical sentiments on displays of nudity.

PROMETHEUS UNCHAINED: ART AND POLITICS

That Prometheus is indeed an apt figure to deliver political messages has been previously shown in our analysis of the nineteenth-century caricature of Karl Marx as the Titan. The

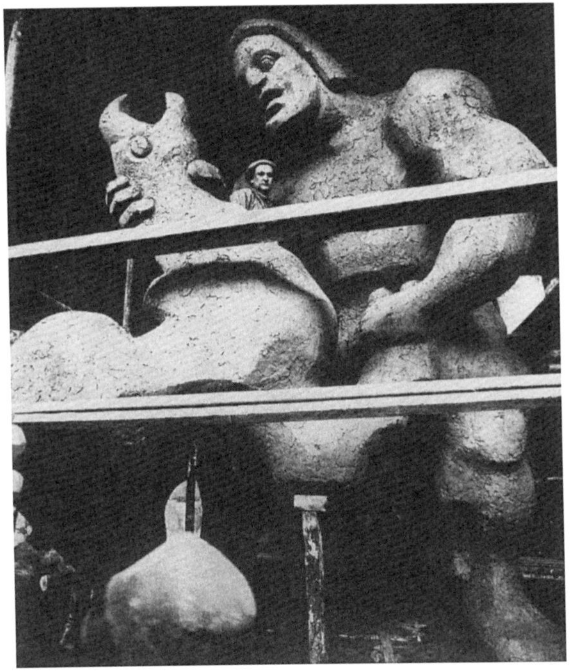

art produced in Europe during and after the Second World War often contained strong political messages. Two European artists, in particular, turned to Prometheus comment on the political situation and to express the effect that the horrors of the War had on them. They both wanted to convey a critique of the war in the figure of Prometheus, but allotted the Titan perfectly opposite roles in their compositions.

The first artist we will examine is the French-Jewish sculptor Jacques Lipchitz (1891-1973). His work illustrates how living situations for Jewish citizens had already started to become untenable before the start of the war. Lipchitz was convinced that one should always strive to rise up against injustice, declaring in an interview that he would always fight for artistic freedom and freedom of expression. His militant approach to the political situation is particularly present in his works that make Prometheus their subject. The artist declared that he wanted to depict a Prometheus 'without his fetters.'

During the 1930s, Lipchitz was commissioned by the French government to create a monumental statue that would be displayed at the opening of the 1937 International Exposition of Art and Technology in Modern Life, which resulted in a remarkable sculpture of the Titan (fig. 13.5). In the work, Prometheus is unchained and has—without any help from Heracles—grabbed the eagle by its throat and strangled it. The eagle makes a formidable opponent, its talons latched into Prometheus' stomach as the Titan tries to pry them out with his free hand. A salient detail is that Prometheus wears a Phrygian cap, a symbol for liberty and democracy in France. By the time the statue was unveiled, it had developed into a powerful political statement. This Prometheus was no longer solely a symbol of mankind conquering ignorance (this was the original meaning given to the statue at its commission), but a direct criticism on German expansionism. The association between the Promethean eagle and the national bird of the German Empire further reinforces this. Lipchitz's statement was praised by proponents of French independence, but heavily criticised by French sympathisers to the fascist regime. Eventually, Lipchitz had to pay a high price for the risk he took with his critical statement: the statue was destroyed in 1938, and the artist had to flee from France. The Prometheus statue only survives now in preparatory sketches and photos that were taken during the International Exposition. Prometheus as a figure of symbolic power remained of interest to Lipchitz for the entirety of his life. After his flight to the United States, Lipchitz revisited the subject many times when reflecting on his experience of the Second World War.

Fig. 13.5 Jaques Lipchitz, photographed while working on his statue of Prometheus for the world fair in Paris, 1937. Prometheus wears a Phrygian cap and has grabbed the screeching eagle by the throat. This imposing plaster statue was 9 meters high and originally stood in Paris, but got destroyed a year after its completion in 1938. (Photograph from: Avigdor W.G. Posèq, 'Jacques Lipchitz's Bird-Headed "Prometheus" and the Related Works', Artibus et Historiae 26 [2005], nr. 52, p. 194)

PROMETHEUS AS SCAPEGOAT: KOKOSCHKA'S ANTI-MATERIALISM

We find an opposite appraisal of Prometheus in the work of Austrian artist Oskar Kokoschka (1886-1980). Kokoschka was determinedly anti-fascit, but had initially not included any political themes in his works. This changed when, to his shock, his art was included in the 1937 Munich exhibition '*Entartete Kunst,*' or art deemed degenerate, organised by the Nazi Party as a direct attack on modernist art. As a counter reaction to his inclusion, Kokoschka produced a series of highly moralising works with political messages in order to make his position more explicit. He was proud to be considered a 'degenerate' artist. In these works, Kokoschka mainly agitated against what he identified as the institutions that were responsible for creating the conditions that allowed for the events of the Second World War to unfold: press, army and technology. He represented this political in his *Prometheus Triptych* , painted in 1950 (fig. 13.6).

The triptych consists of three separate paintings that are intended for joint display (in our index of images, we have first reproduced the entire triptych, followed by close-ups of the separate paintings). In the central panel, we see an apocalyptic scene where, drawing upon biblical imagery, four horsemen signify the end of days. The first three horsemen are representative of the triumvirate of press, technology and army that the artist meant to crit-

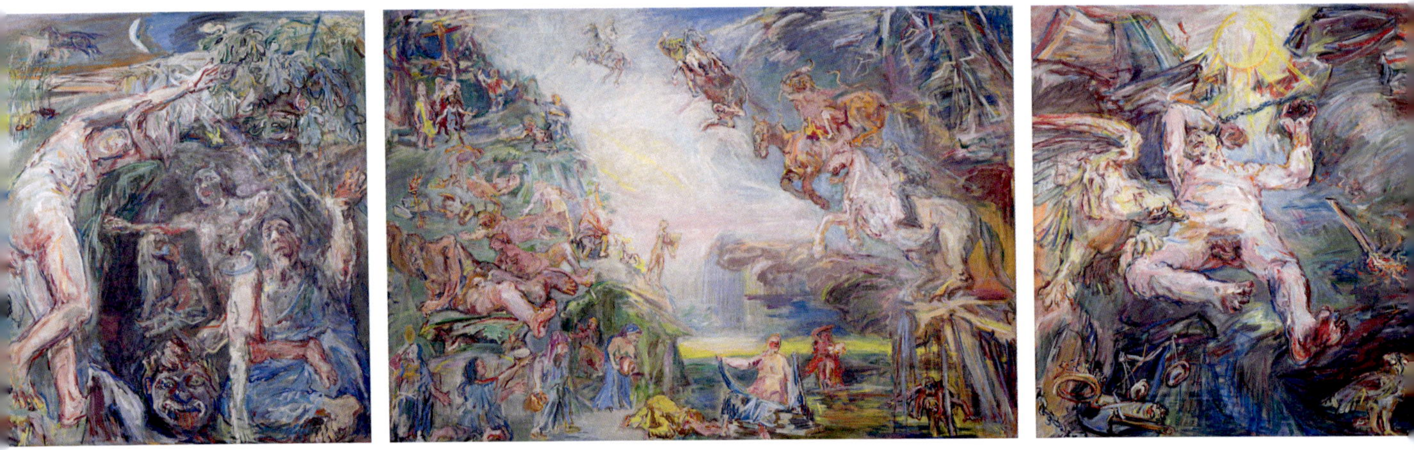

Fig. 13.6 Oskar Kokoschka, Prometheus triptych. On the left panel we see the rape of Persephone, in the middle panel we see a biblical apocalypse with four horsemen. The horsemen stand for press, army and technology, as well as an unidentified fourth horseman. On the right panel we see the punishment of Prometheus, as a metaphor for the adverse effects of unbridled materialism. 1950, oil paint on canvas, 239 × 813 cm, The Samuel Courtauld Trust, The Courtauld Gallery, London, DACS 2003

icize in his work. The horseman on the far right has the face of Moritz Benedikt, editor of the Vienna *Neue freie Presse*, symbolising the institution of the press. The middle horseman symbolises the army, having the face of Kaiser Wilhelm II who holds a weapon up in the air. The third horseman represents science and technology, having the face of Albert Einstein, who Kokoschka blamed for the invention of the nuclear bomb. The mass of figures on the right of the canvas represents the progress and decline of the Judeo-Christian world.

In the left panel, Kokoschka depicts the return of Persephone from the underworld, and in the right, the punishment of Prometheus. He contrasts the verdant world of Persephone with the bare mountain precipice of Prometheus. Kokoschka did not believe that the modern world, which he deemed doomed, could still be saved, least of all through political means. The emblems of the state – a crown, scales and the Nazi fasces (a bound bundle of wooden rods with an axe in the middle that has represented authority since Roman antiquity) – are placed in the right panel where Prometheus receives his punishment. In an essay on his work, Kokoschka called Prometheus a timeless symbol for human arrogance and a cautionary tale of the punishment that awaits us when unbridled faith is put in materialism and progress. In the left panel, he depicts what according to him is the only hope of salvation. Persephone resembles love and the return of nature bringing the world back to life.

Both Kokoschka and Lipchitz spoke out against the National Socialist regime and used Prometheus as a symbol to express their own positions on war and fascism, but ended up doing this in completely opposing ways. Lipchitz showed Prometheus as a militant hero who stood up against oppression, while Kokoschka paints Prometheus as a negative figure representing opposition to what he saw as the only way forward after war: a rejection of progress and materialism, and a renewed focus on love and nature.

In this chapter, we have shown how Prometheus became separated from his strictly mythological origins and was raised to symbol. Various twentieth-century artists made Prometheus a vehicle of meaning to be utilised in the expression of sometimes-conflicting ideologies.

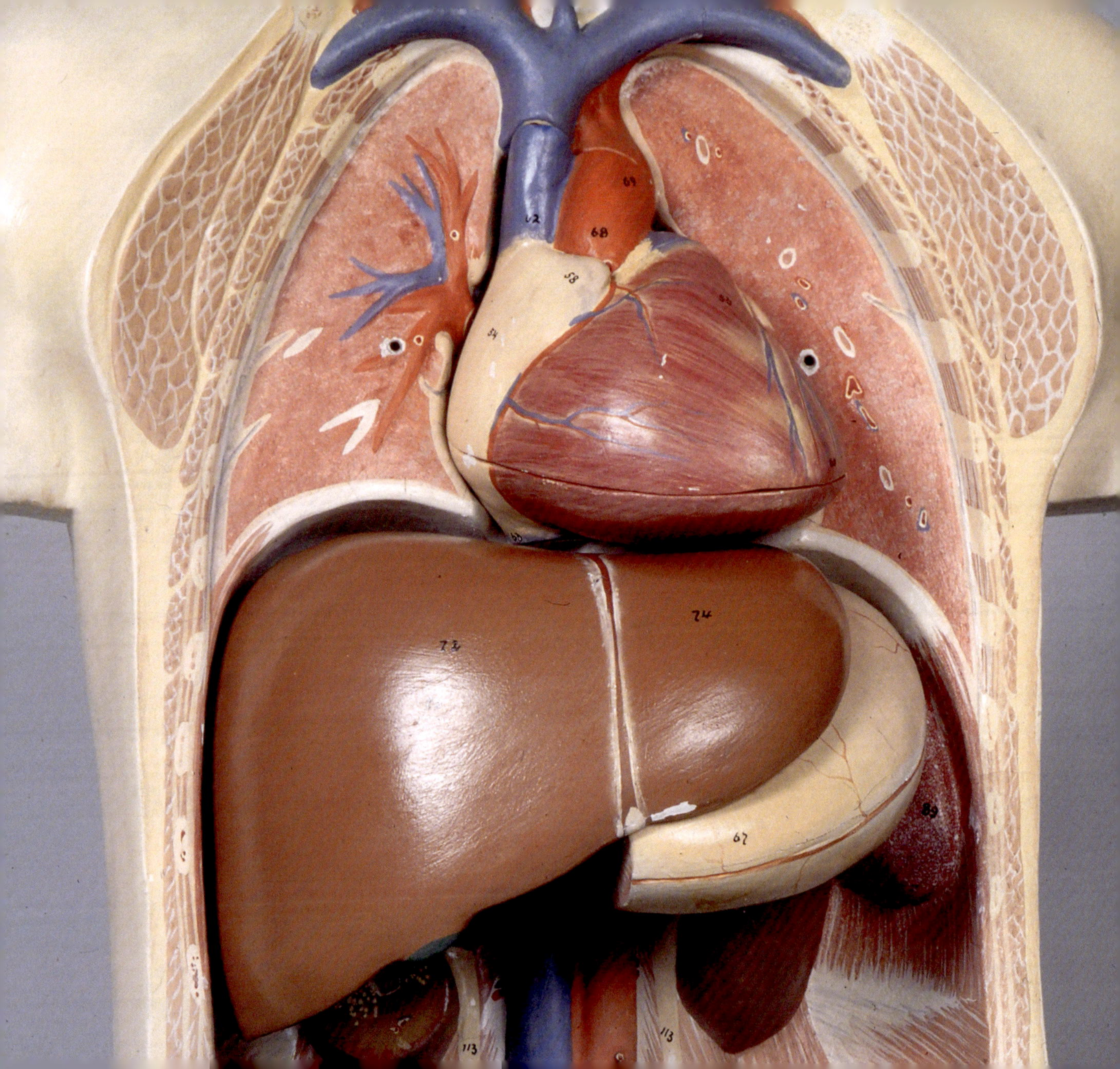
69
68
62
58
54
74
67
89
113
113

14

LIVER SURGERY AND LIVER REGENERATION

In the second half of the nineteenth century, it became possible to operate on patients under general anaesthesia, enabling surgeons to undertake larger and more invasive operations. Most procedures that concern organs in the abdomen were first conceptualised of and performed for the first time in the 1880s. The stomach, the large and small intestine, the appendix and gallbladder could be partially or entirely removed, respectively. The liver, however, was a latecomer. For a long time, the liver was off limits to surgeons due to the high risk of severe bleeding if the organ was cut. This organ contains a dense network of blood vessels—the old belief that blood was produced in the liver was not wholly unfounded (see chapter six). It wasn't until 1952 that the anatomical right half of the organ was successfully removed for the first time in an operation performed in Paris.

Operations on the liver continued to carry a high risk of massive bleeding, which is why only a very few surgeons would risk it. The liver was also akin to a 'black box' that could not be properly depicted with standard x-rays, making it impossible to tell where in the organ a problem was located. It was not until the advent of new imaging techniques like ultrasonography and CT-scans in the 1970s that it became possible to examine the inside

Afb 14.0 Anatomical model that shows the liver in the upper abdominal cavity below the diaphragm, and heart and lungs above the diaphragm. The stomach is for the greater part located behind the liver. Department of Anatomy, Embryology, and Physiology, Amsterdam UMC, location AMC, University of Amsterdam

of the liver. These techniques had tremendous influence on the further development of liver surgery.

Fig. 14.1 Drawing of the hydra that Abraham Trembley discovered in the pools of the estate of Sorghvliet in the Hague. Illustration from Trembley's Mémoires pour servir à l'histoire d'un genre de polypes d'eau douce, *Leiden (Gebr. Verbeek), 1744*

SURGICAL ANATOMY OF THE LIVER

We have seen in the preceding chapters how the anatomical understanding of the liver developed over the course of ten centuries, changing from the five-lobed organ of the Middle Ages (modelled after pig livers) to the accurate depiction of its external properties, as described by Albrecht von Haller in the eighteenth century and depicted in his textbook *Elementa physiologiae corporis humai* (fig. 12.2). Operating on the liver, however, required knowledge of its internal anatomy as well, especially an awareness of the location of major blood vessels, so as to avoid severe bleeding during surgery.

The French surgeon and anatomist Claude Couinaud (1922-2008) first documented the internal anatomy of the liver, closely following this work with a recording of the course of blood vessels and bile ducts throughout the liver. He examined hundreds of livers in the dissecting room, made casts of the network of blood vessels and bile ducts, and created accurate drawings of the positions of all internal structures. Utilising the portal vein and its ramifications, he was able to define distinct areas where the blood supply followed a regular pattern. These areas are called 'segments.' They all possess their own blood supply and bile outlet, which form the basis of the division of the liver into segments. The planes between the segments function as watersheds on where the liver can be cut into without encountering major blood vessels. Couinaud provided every segment with a number so that parts of the liver could be referenced and documented. This division of the liver into segments made it possible to perform operations on the organ by working to the margins of each segment, an important step forward in the development of liver surgery as a discipline (fig. 14.1).

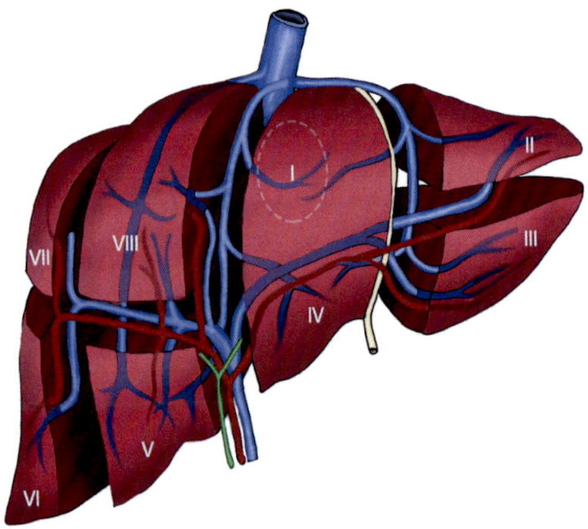

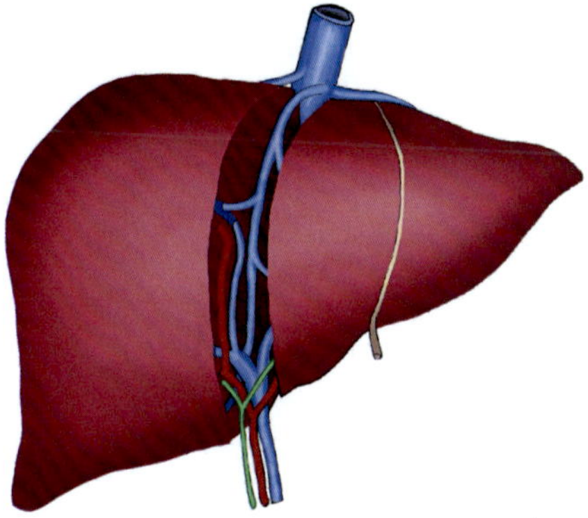

Fig 14.2 a+b It is sometimes necessary to remove the entire (anatomical) right lobe of the liver for a tumor. The liver is cut along the border with the (anatomical) left lobe.

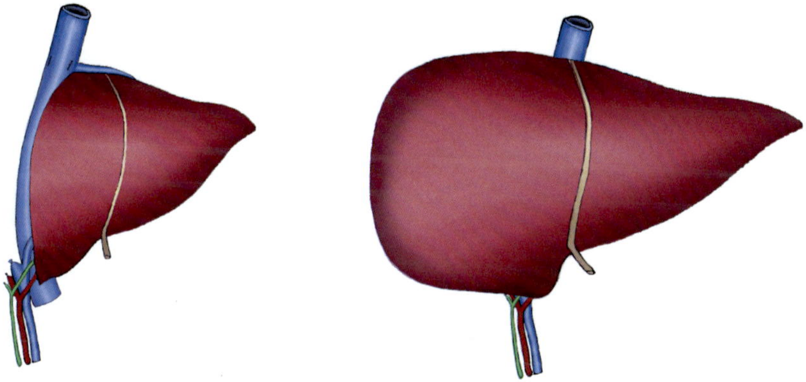

Fig 14.3 a+b The remaining part of the liver grows to almost the original volume of the whole liver in 4-6 weeks, thanks to the regenerative capacity of the liver.

SEVENTY PERCENT OF THE LIVER CAN BE REMOVED

In the present day, most major hospitals perform operations on the liver, the most common of these operations being the removal of tumours. Depending on the size of the growth, a smaller or larger part of the liver is removed in such procedures. For especially complex tumours, or in the occurrence of multiple tumours, it is sometimes necessary to remove the entire right or left lobe of the liver (fig. 14.2 a + b). Thanks to the enormous spare, functional capacity of the liver, it is possible, in healthy livers, to remove up to seventy percent of the liver tissue at once. In response to this loss of liver tissue, the body initiates a fascinating process, where it mass-produces liver cells in order to compensate the lost tissue. This phenomenon is called liver regeneration. Because of this process, the remainder of the liver regrows to close to its original size and weight (fig. 14.3 a + b). The process of liver regeneration is unique in the human body; the liver is the only organ that has this self-regenerating property. We know of such regenerative phenomena in the animal kingdom, such as salamanders, who can regenerate lost tails and the case of the sweet water polyp. When this polyp is cut in two, both halves bloom into two new polyps.

LIVER TRANSPLANTATION

When the liver itself is impacted by illness and its function starts to fail, patients experience a severe decline in their quality of life. The loss of certain liver functions can even lead to life threatening situations, for which there is no other known treatment than a liver transplant. When kidney failure occurs, dialysis can be utilised to take on some of the blood filtering properties of the kidneys, but for the liver, such an artificial replacement of its essential tasks does not exist. Liver transplantation is a complex procedure where the entire liver is removed and replaced with the liver of an organ donor. The first successful liver transplants were executed in 1960 in Denver (US) and Cambridge (UK). At this moment – entirely in the Promethean spirit – a new frontier was crossed and a perspective found for the development of a viable treatment for patients with chronic liver disease.

In the case of acute liver failure, there is a temporary solution that makes use of the regenerative properties of the liver, where a donor liver is transplanted without the removal of the patient's own liver. The transplanted liver will take on a role as 'auxiliary engine,' while the patient's damaged liver has the opportunity to regenerate itself. After

REGENERATION OF THE HYDRA POLYP

Abraham Trembley (1710-1784) was a Swiss physicist who, in 1736, was appointed by Count Willem Bentinck van Rhoon to instruct Bentinck's two sons in his mansion at the Sorghvliet estate (now called the Catshuis) near The Hague. Trembley took the two boys, aged three and six, to the ponds of the estate as part of his teachings in natural history, to instruct them on the life forms that could be found in their waters. In these ponds, he discovered a curious small creature, which he was uncertain whether it was plant or animal. He called it a 'polyp' and kept these polyps in jars filled with pond water to investigate them further. The boys aided him in his research by using nets to catch polyps and together, they looked at the curious little creatures through a microscope. Trembley saw and described that each polyp possessed a head and a variable number of tentacles and that, when he cut off the head or an arm, a new head or arm would sprout from its original location on the body. Even when Trembley bisected a polyp, both halves grew into two new polyps, complete with seven or more tentacles. This fascinating discovery of the regenerative properties of fresh water polyps was revolutionary at the time, and became the talk of famed scientific salons in Western Europe

Seeing the resemblance between his polyps and the mythological self-regenerating monster the Hydra of Lerna, Trembley christened these polyps 'Hydra.' The Hydra is now classified as a freshwater anemone under the name *Hydra viridis* (green hydra) or *Chlorophyta viridissima*. Trembley's experiments on the Hydra of Sorghvliet introduced the concept of regeneration as a form of self-preservation to the scientific public.

Image of a hydra that Abraham Trembley discovered in the ponds of the Sorghvliet estate in The Hague. Illustration from Trembley's Mémoires pour servir à l'histoire d'un genre de polypes d'eau douce, *Leiden (Gebr. Verbeek), 1744*

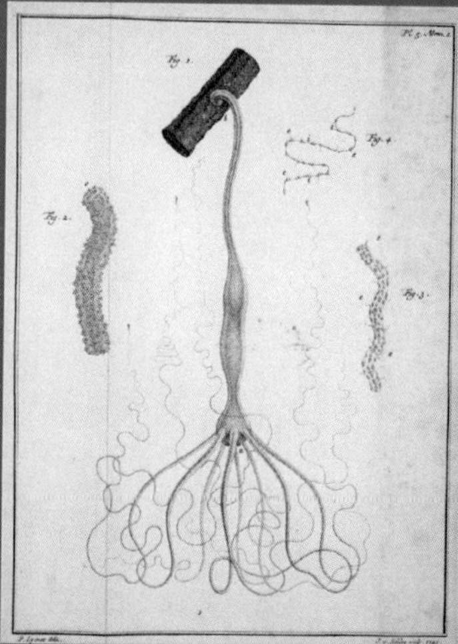

liver functions have normalised, the transplanted liver has fulfilled its purpose and can be removed in a second operation. All of this would be impossible without liver regeneration.

LIVER REGENERATION, THE TRUSTED ALLY OF THE LIVER SURGEON

The regenerative properties of the liver make it possible to remove large parts of the organ. This property is liberally relied upon in the surgical treatment of tumours of the liver. Thus, liver regeneration is an important ally to the liver surgeon. The myth of Prometheus, in which the liver that was consumed by the eagle that tortured the Titan during the day regenerates by night, has always captivated liver surgeons and liver specialists. The salient correspondence between the myth and anatomical reality could lead one to speculate whether the ancient Greeks might have been subconsciously aware of these regenerative properties when writing their myths.

PROMETHEUS: SYMBOL OF LIVER REGENERATION

This correspondence has made Prometheus the symbol of the regenerative properties of the liver in the medical field. It is, however, very unlikely that the ancient Greeks were aware of these properties and that they are inexhaustible. The gods, of which the Titan Prometheus was one, were immortal and so were their bodies. That a divine liver was thus imperishable, and could regenerate when part of it had been lost, corresponded with their Olympic view of immortality and belief in the possibility of eternal renewal of body parts. In the mythology of the ancient Greeks, more instances of the regeneration of body parts can be found. One such example would be the Hydra of Lerna, a poisonous serpentine monster with nine heads that haunted the Lake of Lerna near Argolis, and the aforementioned namesake of Trembley's polyp (fig. 14.4). When the legendary hero Herakles fought the creature, he found that for each head he cut off, two new ones would grow in its place. He was only able to defeat the Hydra with the

Fig 14.4 Etruscan amphora depicting the Hydra of Lerna, a serpent monster with nine heads. Heracles went into battle with the monster, but everytime he cut off one of its heads, two heads grew back! 530-500 BC. (44.6 × 38 × 33.4 cm), J. Paul Getty Museum, Los Angeles CA

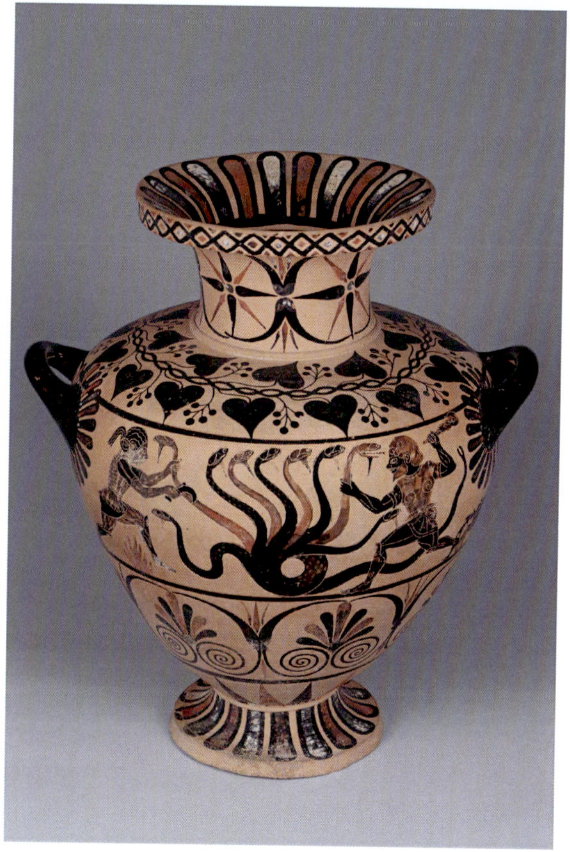

assistance of his partner, Iolaus, who would cauterize the stump of the neck with a torch before the new heads had the chance to sprout.

In Greek mythology, Prometheus was punished by the supreme god Zeus for giving humanity the Olympic fire with which they learned to think and feel, providing them with ingenuity and ambition. He was chained to a cliff in the Caucasus, where he was visited daily by an eagle who ate part of his liver. At night, however, his liver grew back. Gods were immortal and so were their bodies including their organs and therefore, the liver after sustaining loss, would be renewed. We now know that the liver can regenerate after part of it has been removed, and although the ancient Greeks were not aware of this self-regenerating process, they arrived at the same conclusion. That liver regeneration still reminds us of Prometheus is evidence of how powerful the imagery of his tragic fate still is in our collective consciousness – a fate that from antiquity to the present day inspired both scientists and artists to push forward and to create.

ACKNOWLEDGEMENTS

The research that resulted in this book was inspired by the article 'Prometheus and Liver Regeneration; the Dissection of a Myth' published in *The Netherlands Journal of Medicine* (2018; 162; D2882) and written by Thomas van Gulik and others. We want to thank Hugo Koning (Faculty of Humanities, University of Leiden) for his contributions to this article, where he introduced us to Prometheus and his myth.

We thank Bouke van der Meer (Faculty of Archaeology, University of Leiden) for his contributions to the chapter on the Etruscan liver of Piacenza. We also want to express our gratitude to the firm J. Korver (Abcoude) for supplying us with sheep livers for our own observation.

We extend our gratitude to Caroline LaPorte-Burns for her assistance in editing this English copy as well as her insight on an article that will be based on this book.

We thank the Board of Directors of the Amsterdam UMC for supporting this project.

ON THE AUTHORS

Julia van Rosmalen studied art history at the Courtauld institute of Art in London

Merel van Gulik studied classics and Italian language and culture at the University of Amsterdam

Belle van Rosmalen is a PhD candidate at the Department of Surgery at the Amsterdam University Medical Centers, University of Amsterdam

Thomas van Gulik is Em. Professor of Surgery at the Amsterdam University Medical Centers, University of Amsterdam

BIBLIOGRAPHY

1 - The Prometheus myth

Fry, S., *Mythos*. London: Michael Joseph/Penguin Random House 2017

Lamb, W.R.M. (red. en vert.), *Plato. Laches, Protagoras, Meno, Euthydemus*. Cambridge, MA: Harvard University Press 1924

Most, G. W. (red. en vert.), *Hesiod. Theogony, Works and Days, Testimonia*. Cambridge, MA: Harvard University Press 2018

Sommerstein, A. H. (red. and vert.), *Aeschylus. Persians, Seven against Thebes, Suppliants, Prometheus Bound*. Cambridge, MA: Harvard University Press 2009

2 - The depiction of prometheus in classical antiquity

Alexandridou, Alexandra-Fani, *The Early Black-Figured Pottery of Attika in Context (C. 630-570 BCE)*, Leiden: Brill 2011

Beazley, J.D., 'Prometheus Fire-Lighter', *American Journal of Archaeology*, 43 (okt.-dec. 1939), nr. 4, p. 618-639

Dawkins, R.M. (red.), *The Sanctuary of Artemis Orthia at Sparta*, London, 1929, pl. 100, p. 209-210

Dougherty, Carol, *Prometheus*, London: Routledge 2006
Furtwängler, A., 'Prometheus', *Archäologische Zeitung*, 43 (1885), p. 223-228
Gantz, Timothy, *Early Greek Myth A Guide to Literary and Artistic Sources*, Baltimore: Johns Hopkins University Press 1996
Grummond, Nancy De, Simon Thomson en Larissa Bonfante, *The Religion of the Etruscans*, Austin: University of Texas Press 2006, p. 20, afb. II.6
Hesiod / Glenn W. Most (red.), *Hesiod Revised*, Cambridge (MA): Harvard University Press 2018
Puma, Richard Daniel de, en Christopher Lightfoot, *Etruscan Art in the Metropolitan Museum of Art*, nr. 6.40, New Haven/London: The Metropolitan Museum of Art 2013, p. 173, 200-201
Richter, Gisela M.A., 'Prometheus', *The British Museum Quarterly*, 32 (herfst 1967), nrs. 1-2, p. 6-8
Smith, R.R.R., 'The Imperial Reliefs from the Sebasteion at Aphrodisias', *The Journal of Roman Studies*, 77 (1987), p. 88-138
Terzaghi, N., 'Monumenti di Prometeo', in: *Studi e Materiali Archeologia e Numismatica*, dl. 3, Milaan 1905, p. 199-215

3 - The liver according to the ancient Greeks and the etruscans

MacIntosh Turfa, J., Gettys, S. 'The skill of the Etruscan Haruspex. A biological basis for successful divination?', *BABESCH*, 84 (2009), p. 41-52
Mani, N., *Die historischen Grundlagen der Leberforschung*, dl. 1: *Die Vorstellungen über Anatomie, Physiologie und Pathologie der Leber in der Antike*, Bazel/Stuttgart 1965 (2nd edition)
Meer, L.B. van der, *The bronze liver of Piacenza*, Amsterdam (Uitgeverij J.C. Gieben), 1987
Michel, C., 'Ein Manuskript in Form einer Schafsleber', in: Andreas Janke (red.), *Manuskript des Monat*, 10 (2015), SFB 950: Hamburg. http://www.manuscript-cultures.uni-hamburg.de/mom/2015_10_mom.html

Riva, M.A., E. Riva, M. Spicci, M. Strazzabosco, M. Giovannini, G. Cesana, '"The city of Hepar": Rituals, gastronomy, and politics at the origins of the modern names for the liver', *Journal of Hepatology*, 55 (2010), p. 1132-1136
Tiniakos, D.G., A. Kandilis, S.A. Geller, 'Tityus: a forgotten myth of liver regeneration, *Journal of Hepatology*, 53 (2010), p. 357-361

4 - The haruspex and Hepatoscopy

Gulik, T.M. van, H. Lang, 'Isolated resection of segment 1 of the liver', *Digestive Surgery*, 22 (2005), p. 143-148
Lulof P.S., Kampen I. van (red.), 'Etrusken; Vrouwen van aanzien, mannen met macht', WBOOKS, 2011.
MacIntosh Turfa, J., Gettys, S. 'The skill of the Etruscan Haruspex. A biological basis for successful divination?', *BABESCH*, 84 (2009), p. 41-52
Meer, L.B. van der, *The bronze liver of Piacenza*, Amsterdam (Uitgeverij J.C. Gieben), 1987

5 - Prometheus in the Middle Ages

Balty, Janine, Françoise Briquel Chatonnet, 'Nouvelles mosaïques inscrites d'Osrhoène', in: *Monuments et mémoires de la Fondation Eugène Piot*, Paris 2000, dl. 79, p. 31-72
Baratte, François, Catherine Metzger, *Musée du Louvre: catalogue des sarcophages en pierre d'époques romaine et paléochrétienne*, Paris (Éditions de la Réunion des musées nationaux), 1985, p. 115-118
Berg, B., 'Alcestis and Hercules in the Catacomb of via Latina', in: *Vigiliae Christianae*, 48 (1994), nr. 3, p. 219-234
Bowerstock, G.W., 'Notes on the New Edessene Mosaic of Prometheus', *Hyperboreus*, 7 (2001, ed. 2002), fasc. 1-2, p. 411-416
Bowerstock, G.W., *Mosaics as History: The Near East from Late Antiquity to Islam*, Harvard MA, (Harvard University Press), 2006

Elsner, J., 'Archaeologies and Agendas: Reflections on Late Ancient Jewish Art and Early Christian Art', *The Journal of Roman Studies*, 93 (2003), p. 114-128

Finney, P.C., *The invisible God: The earliest Christians on Art*, Oxford (Oxford University Press), 1994

Raggio, Olga, 'The Myth of Prometheus', *Journal of the Courtauld and Warburg Institutes*, 21 (1958), nr. 1, p. 44-62

Spera, L., 'The Christianization of Space along the via Appia: Changing Landscape in the Suburbs of Rome', *American Journal of Archaeology*, 107 (2003), nr. 1, p. 23-43

Tertullianus, *Apologeticum*, boek XVIII

Wyche, Rose-Marie, 'An Archaeology of Memory: the "Reinvention" of Roman Sarcophagi in Provence during the Middle Ages', Phd Thesis, University of Oxford, 2013

6 - The liver in the in the Middle Ages, according to Galenus

Apocalypse, Wellcome Library, London, MS49, fol. 36 v., ca.1420

Cambridge, Library of Gonville and Caius College, MS. 190/223, fol. 5r. Late 12th century. Image: Courtesy of the Master and Fellows of Gonville and Caius College, Cambridge

Chen, T.S., P.S. Chen, 'Understanding the liver. A History', in: *Contributions in medical history*, 14, Westport CT/London (Greenwood Press), 1984

Mani, N., *Die historischen Grundlagen der Leberforschung*, dl. 2: *Die Geschichte der Leberforschung von Galen bis Claude Bernard, Schwabe en Co*, Bazel/Stuttgart, 1967 (1st edition)

McCall, Taylor, 'Disembodied: Additional MS.8785 and the tradition of human organ depictions in medieval art and medicine', eBLJ (Electronic British Library Journal) 2018, Article 8

Temkin, O., Straus W.L., 'Galen's dissection of the liver and of the muscles moving the forearm (vert. van de 'Anatomical procedures'), *Bulletin of the History of Medicine*, 19 (1946), p. 167-176

7 - Prometheus in the renaissance

Alpatov, M.V., S. Bradshaw, 'Allegory and Symbolism in Italian Renaissance Painting', *Diogenes* (1971), 19 (76), p. 1-25

Aston, Margaret (red.), *The panorama of the Renaissance*, New York (Harry N. Abraham Publishers), 1996

Barsella, S., 'The Myth of Prometheus in Giovanni Boccaccio's "Decameron"'sd, *MLN*, 119 (2004), nr. 1, p. 120-141

Boccaccio, Giovanni, *Genealogia Deorum Gentilium*, Rome (appresso Francesco Lorenzini da Turino), 1564 (copy in the National Central Library in Rome)

Cassirer, Ernst, *The individual and the cosmos in Renaissance philosophy*, New York (Harper & Row) 1964

Colvin, S., *A Florentine Picture Chronicle*, London (Bernard Quaritch), 1898

Fermor, Sharon, *Piero di Cosimo: fiction, invention, and fantasìa*, London (Reaktion Books), 1993

Geronimus, Dennis, *Piero Di Cosimo: Visions Beautiful and Strange*, Yale (Yale University Press), 2006

Lüdemann, P., 'Vom Ursprung der Menschheit ins Florenz der Medici: Piero di Cosimos Prometheus-Tafeln in München und Straßburg', *Marburger Jahrbuch für Kunstwissenschaft*, 37 (2010), p. 121-149;

Panofsky, E., 'The Early History of Man in a Cycle of Paintings by Piero di Cosimo', *Journal of the Warburg Institute*, 1 (1937), nr. 1, p. 12-30;

Panofsky, Erwin, *Studies in iconology: humanistic themes in the art of the renaissance*, [s.l.] London (Routledge), 2019

Raggio, Olga, 'The Myth of Prometheus', *Journal of the Courtauld and Warburg Institutes* 21 (1958), nr. 1, p. 44-62

The decorative program of the studiolo of Francesco I can be found at: http://museicivicifiorentini.comune.fi.it/en/palazzovecchio/visitamuseo/studiolo_francesco_i.htm

8 - The liver in the Renaissance as described by Reisch, Vesalius and Da Vinci

Clayton, M., R. Philo, *Leonardo da Vinci, Anatomist*, London (Royal Collection Trust), 2017
Hee (red.), R. van, *Art of Vesalius*, Antwerp/Apeldoorn (Garant), 2014
Lindeboom, G.A., *Andreas Vesalius and his opus magnum. A biographical sketch and an introduction to the Fabrica*, Nieuwendijk (De Forel BV), 1975
Lint, J.G. de, *Atlas van de Geschiedenis der Geneeskunde. I. De Ontleedkunde*, Amsterdam (S.L. van Looy, Menno Herzberger), 1925
Nykonenko, A., P. Vavra, P. Zonca, 'Pecularities of pig and human liver', *Experimental and Clinical Transplantation*, 15 (2017), nr. 1, p. 21-26
Reisch, Gregor, *Margarita Philosophica*, Freiburg 1503
Rifkin, B.A., Ackerman, M.J., Menselijke anatomie (van de renaissance tot het digitale tijdperk), Roeselare (Roularta Books), 2006
Vesalius, A., *De humani corporis fabrica libri septem.*, Bazel (Oporinus), 1543 / Facsimile edition Nieuwendijk (De Forel BV), 1975

9 - Prometheus in the Baroque

Alpers, Svetlana, *The Art of Describing: Dutch Art in the Seventeenth Century*, Chicago (University of Chicago Press), 1983
Bikker, J., 'Lucian's Prometheus as a Source for Jordaens and van Baburen', *Simiolus: Netherlands Quarterly for the History of Art*, 31 (2004), nr. 1/2, p. 47-53
Carl, Klaus, *Baroque Art*, New York (Parkstone International), 2014
Dempsey, C., 'Euanthes Redivivus: Rubens's Prometheus Bound', *Journal of the Warburg and Courtauld Institutes*, 30 (1967), p. 420-425
Hanson, Julie V., 'Resurrecting Death: Anatomical Art in the Cabinet of Dr. Frederik Ruysch', *Art Bulletin*, 78 (dec. 1996), nr. 4, p. 663-679
Hauser, Arnold, *The Social History of Art: Renaissance, Mannerism and Baroque*, London (Routledge), 1990

Held, Julius S., 'Prometheus Bound', *Philadelphia Museum of Art Bulletin*, 59 (1963), (279), p. 17-32
IJpma, Frank, Van Gulik, Thomas, *Amsterdamse anatomische lessen ontleed*, Amsterdam (Boom), 2013
Jones, Amelia, Robert S. Nelson, Richard Schiff (red.), 'Body', in: *Critical Terms for Art History*, Chicago (University of Chicago Press), 2003, p. 251-266
Kimball, F., 'Rubens' Prometheus', *The Burlington Magazine*, 94 (1952), (588), p. 67-70
Langdon, Helen, 'The Demosthenes of Painting. Salvator Rosa and the 17th century Sublime', in: *Translations of the Sublime*, Leiden (Martinus Nijhoff/Brill), 2012, p. 163-185
Raggio, Olga, 'The Myth of Prometheus', *Journal of the Courtauld and Warburg Institutes*, 21 (1958), nr. 1, p. 44-62

9 (insert) - The wounds of christ and prometheus – two of a kind?

Barb, A.A., 'The Wound in Christ's Side', *Journal of the Warburg and Courtauld Institutes*, 34 (1971), p. 320-321
Bynum, Caroline W., *Jesus As Mother: Studies in the Spirituality of the High Middle Ages*, Berkeley MA (University of California Press), 1984
Ehrman, Bart D., Zlatko Pleše, *The Apocryphal Gospels: Texts and Translations*, New York (Oxford University Press), 2011
Gurewich, Vladimir, 'Observations on the Iconography of the Wound in Christ's Side, with Special Reference to Its Position', *Journal of the Warburg and Courtauld Institutes*, 20 (1957), no. 3/4, p. 358-362
Gurewich, Vladimir, 'Rubens and the Wound in Christ's Side. A Postscript', *Journal of the Warburg and Courtauld Institutes*, 26 (1963), no. 3/4, p. 358-358
Kirkham, Anne, Cordelia Warr, *Wounds in the Middle Ages*, Farnham (Ashgate Publishing Ltd), 2014
Millet, Gabriel, *Recherches Sur L'iconographie De L'évangile Aux 14., 15., Et 16. Siècles:*

D'après Les Monuments De Mistra, De La Macédoine Et Du Mont Athos : Dessins De Sophie Millet, Paris (E. de Boccard), 1960

Schechter, Solomon, Ludwig Blau, M. Seligsohn, 'LIVER (כבד)', in: Isidore Singer (red.), *The Jewish Encyclopedia: A Descriptive Record of the History, Religion, Literature, and Customs of the Jewish People from the Earliest Times to the Present Day*, New York (Funk and Wagnalls), 1901, dl. 8, p. 140-141

10 - The liver in the Baroque, according to van der Spiegel, Glisson and Bidloo

Broos, P., *Anatomia; de ontdekking van het menselijk lichaam in de Lage Landen (16e-18e eeuw)*, Antwerp (Davidsfonds & WPG Uitgevers België NV) / Amsterdam (AUP), 2017

IJpma, F.F.A., van Gulik T.M., 'Bidloo's and De Lairesse's early illustrations of the anatomy of the arm (1690): a successful collaboration between a prominent physician and a talented artist', *Journal of Hand Surgery (European Volume)*, 38 (2013), nr. 1, p. 94-99

Lindeboom, G.A., 'Adriaan van den Spiegel (1578-1625): hoogleraar in de ontleed- en heelkunde te Padua', in: *Nieuwe Nederlandse Bijdragen tot de Geschiedenis der Geneeskunde en der Natuurwetenschappen*, nr. 2, Amsterdam (Rodopi), 1978

Spiegel, A. van den, *De Humani Corporis Fabrica Libri Decem*, Frankfurt 1632

Wellcome Collection, L0032415

Gulik, T.M. van, 'Francis Glisson's anatomy of the liver and biliary tract', *Hepato-gastroenterology* (1990), 37, p. 530-531

Guest, R.V., Margocsy S., Wigmore S.J., 'Govert Bidloo's liver: human symmetry reflected', *Lancet*, 383 (2014), p. 688-689

11 - Prometheus and modernity

Anonymus, 'Jean Jacques Pradier', *The Illustrated Magazine of Art*, 2 (1853), nr. 7, p. 56-58

Corbeau-Parsons, Caroline, *Prometheus in the Nineteenth Century: From Myth to Symbol*, Leeds (Taylor and Francis), 2013

Curran, Stuart, 'The Political Prometheus', *Studies in Romanticism*, 25 (1986), nr. 3, p. 429-455
Goethe, Johann W. von, Manfred Meurer, *Prometheus*, Stratford (Book Stage), 2004
Indirkas, Zuhre, 'Transformations of Prometheus throughout the Ages', *International Journal of the Humanities*, 9 (2012), nr. 8, p. 109-128
Junker, Patricia, 'Thomas Cole's "Prometheus Bound". An Allegory for the 1840s', *American Art Journal*, 31 (2000), nr. 1/2, p. 33-55
Moriarty, Michael, 'Structures of Cultural Production in Nineteenth-Century France', in: Collier, Peter, Robert Lethbridge (red.), *Artistic Relations. Literature and the Visual Arts in Nineteenth-Century France*, New Haven/London (Yale University Press), 1994, p. 15-29
Shelley, Percy B., Alex Gutteling (vert.), *Prometheus Ontboeid. Een Lyrisch Drama in Vier Bedrijven*, Amsterdam (Wereldbibliotheek), 1910.
Smith, David Norman, 'Prometheus Unchained Marx's Abolitionism', *Dialectical Anthropology*, 39 (2015), nr. 2, p. 211-214
Williams, Raymond, 'The romantic artist', in: *Culture and society 1780-1950*, Columbia (Columbia University Press), 1958, p. 48-64

11 (insert) - Mary Shelley's Frankenstein: or the modern Prometheus

Foertsch, Jacqueline. 'The Right, the Wrong, and the Ugly: Teaching Shelley's Several "Frankensteins"', *College English*, 63 (2001), nr. 6, p. 697-671Horton, Robert, 'The monster's place', in: *Frankenstein*, New York/Chichester (Columbia University Press), 2014, p. 84-96
Hustis, Harriet, 'Responsible creativity and the "modernity" of Mary Shelley's Prometheus', *SEL Studies in English Literature 1500-1900*, 43 (2003), nr. 4, p. 845-858
Shelley, Mary W., *Frankenstein* [1818], Atlanta GA (Intervisual Books), 2010
Sherwin, Paul, 'Frankenstein: Creation as Catastrophe', *PMLA*, 96 (1981), nr. 5, p. 883-903

12 - The liver in the Enlightenment

Bernard, Claude, *Introduction à l'étude de la medicine experimentale*, Paris (Librairie Joseph Gibert), 1865

Chen, T.S., P.S. Chen, 'Understanding the liver; A History', *Contributions in medical history*, number 14. Westport CT/Connecticut (Greenwood Press), London 1984

Haller, Albrecht von, *Elementa physiologiae corporis humani*, Lausanne (Marci-Michael Bousquet), 1557-1566

Hintzsche, E., *Albrecht von Hallers Briefe an Auguste Tissot*, Bern/Stuttgart/Wenen (Verlag Hans Huber), 1977

Lindeboom, G.A., *Haller in Holland. Dagboek*, Delft (Koninklijke Nederlandsche Gist- en Spiritusfabriek NV), 1958

Mani, N., *Die historischen Grundlagen der Leberforschung*. Dl. 2: *Die Geschichte der Leberforschung von Galen bis Claude Bernard, Schwabe en Co*, Bazel/Stuttgart (Schwabe & Co.), 1967 (1st edition 1965)

13 - The 20th century Prometheus

Macaulay-Lewis, Matthew McGowan (red.), *Classical New York: Discovering Greece and Rome in Gotham*, New York (Fordham University Press), 2018, p. 140-160

Mesquita, Nicholas Bueno de, 'Karl Kraus, Oskar Kokoschka and "The Prometheus Triptych"', *The Burlington Magazine*, 151 (2009), nr. 1276, p. 444-452

Mola, Paola (red.), *Brancusi. The White Work*, tent.cat. The Peggy Guggenheim Collection, Venice, 2005

Mullaly, Terence, 'Impact of Kokoschka', *RSA Journal*, 138 (1990), nr. 5410, p. 709

Posèq, Avigdor W.G., 'Jacques Lipchitz's Bird-Headed "Prometheus" and the Related Works', *Artibus Et Historiae*, 26 (2005), nr. 52, p. 189-199

Rowell, Margit, 'František Kupka: Prometheus', *The Print Collector's Newsletter*, 6 (1975), nr. 5, p. 129-132

Scott, David W., 'Orozco's Prometheus: Summation, Transition, Innovation', *College Art*

Journal, 17 (1957), nr. 1, p. 2-18
Simard, Jared A., 'The Titans of Rockefeller Center: Prometheus and Atlas', in: Elizabeth Theinhardt, Markéta, 'La «gamme jaune» de František Kupka: un exemple de synesthésie', *Revue Des études Slaves*, 74 (2002), nr. 1, p. 97-103
Vanechkina, I.L., Galeyev B.M., ' "Prometheus": Scriabin Kandinsky', *Leonardo*, 31 (1998), nr. 3, p. 183-184
Wright, Barnaby, 'Oskar Kokoschka at Work on "The Prometheus Triptych": Unseen Photographs by Lee Miller', *The Burlington Magazine*, 151 (2009), nr. 1276, p. 453-455

14 - Liver surgery and liver regeneration

Chen, T.S.N., P.S.Y. Chen, 'The myth of Prometheus and the liver', *Journal of the Royal Society of Medicine*, 87 (1994), p. 754-755
Couinaud, C., *Surgical anatomy of the liver revisited*, Paris (personal edition), 1989
Gulik, T.M. van, Gulik, M.M. van, Koning, H.H., 'Prometheus en leverregeneratie; de ontleding van een mythe', *Nederlands Tijdschrift voor Geneeskunde* (2018), 162: D2882
Lortat-Jacob, J.L., Robert, H.G., Hépatectomie droite réglée, La Presse Medicale (1952), 60: 549-551
Nederlandse Leverpatienten Vereniging (Dutch association for liver patients), https://www.leverpatientenvereniging.nl/levertransplantatie
Power, C., Rasko, J.E.J., '"Whither Prometheus" liver? Greek myth and the science of regeneration', *Annals of Internal Medicine*, 149 (2008), p. 421-426
Terpstra OT, Schalm SW, Weimar W, et al. Auxiliary partial liver transplantation for end-stage chronic liver disease. N Engl J Med (1988), 319: 1507-11
Taub, R., 'Liver regeneration: from myth to mechanism', *Nature Reviews Molecular Cell Biology* (2004), nr. 5, p. 836-847
Tiniakos, D.G., Kandilis A., Geller S.A., 'Tityus: a forgotten myth of liver regeneration', *Journal of Hepatology*, 53 (2010), p. 357-361

14 (insert) - Regeneration of the Hydra polyp

Lenhoff, S.G., Lenhoff, H.M., *Hydra and the Birth of Experimental Biology – 1744. Abraham Trembley's Memoires Concerning the Polyps*, Pacific Grove CA (The Boxwood Press), 1986

INDEX

First published in 2022 by Amsterdam University Press Ltd.

Published 2025 by Routledge
4 Park Square, Milton Park, Abingdon, Oxon OX14 4RN
605 Third Avenue, New York, NY 10158

Routledge is an imprint of the Taylor & Francis Group, an informa business

ISBN: 9789463723091 (hbk)
ISBN: 9781041184751 (pbk)
ISBN: 9781003702078 (ebk)
NUR 640, 680

Graphic Design Bart van den Tooren
Translation Julia van Rosmalen

DOI: 10.5117/9789463723091

For Product Safety Concerns and Information please contact our EU representative: GPSR@taylorandfrancis.com
Taylor & Francis Verlag GmbH, Kaufingerstraße 24, 80331 München, Germany

TotalPos Not Define

For Product Safety Concerns and Information please contact our EU representative GPSR@taylorandfrancis.com Taylor & Francis Verlag GmbH, Kaufingerstraße 24, 80331 München, Germany

Printed and bound by CPI Group (UK) Ltd, Croydon, CR0 4YY
11/09/2026
02215149-0001